Natural Hormone Solutions

Other titles in the
Women's Edge Health Enhancement Guide
series:

Busy Woman's Cookbook
Energy for Everything
Fight Fat
Food Smart
Foolproof Weight Loss
Get Well, Stay Well
Growing Younger
Herbs That Heal
Natural Remedies
The Inner Journey
Total Body Toning

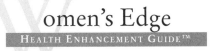

Women's Edge

HEALTH ENHANCEMENT GUIDE™

Natural Hormone Solutions

Secrets to Conquering Stress, Weight, Aging, Menopause, and More

By Elizabeth Shimer, Marie Elaina Suszynski, and the Editors of

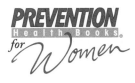

PREVENTION

Health Books®

for Women

RODALE

NOTICE

This book is intended as a reference volume only, not as a medical manual. The information given here is designed to help you make informed decisions about your health. It is not intended as a substitute for any treatment that may have been prescribed by your doctor. If you suspect that you have a medical problem, we urge you to seek competent medical help.

Beginning on page 169, you will find safe use guidelines for supplements, herbs, or essential oils recommended in this book that will help you use these remedies safely and wisely.

Mention of specific companies, organizations, or authorities in this book does not imply endorsement by the publisher, nor does mention of specific companies, organizations, or authorities in the book imply that they endorse the book.

Internet addresses and telephone numbers given in this book were accurate at the time the book went to press.

© 2001 Rodale Inc.

Illustrations by Shawn Banner, Judy Newhouse, Tom Ward
Cover photographs © by Don Farrall/PhotoDisc, Hilmar, Rita Maas

Printed in the United States of America
Rodale Inc. makes every effort to use acid-free ♾, recycled paper ♻.

The hormonal health questionnaire on page 8 was reprinted from *Balance Hormones Naturally* by Kate Neil and Patrick Holford. © 1999 by The Crossing Press.
The chart of thyroid function tests on page 38 is © 2001 by Mary Shomon, About, Inc. Used by permission of About, Inc., which can be found on the Web at www.About.com. All rights reserved.
The assessment quiz for human growth hormone on page 72 was adapted from *Grow Young with HGH*, by Ronald Klatz, M.D., president of the American Academy of Anti-Aging Medicine, with Carol Kahn. © 1998 by HarperPerennial.

Library of Congress Cataloging-in-Publication Data

Shimer, Elizabeth.
    Natural hormone solutions : secrets to conquering stress, weight, aging, menopause, and more / by Elizabeth Shimer, Marie Elaina Suszynski, and the editors of Prevention Health Books for Women.
        p.   cm. — (Women's edge health enhancement guide)
    Includes index.
    ISBN 1–57954–350–2 hardcover
    1. Hormones—Popular works.   2. Women—Health and hygiene.   3. Women—Diseases—Endocrine aspects.
    I. Suszynski, Marie Elaina.   II. Prevention Health Books for Women.   III. Title.   IV. Series.
    QP571 .S54   2001
    615'.36'082—dc21   2001001129

Distributed to the book trade by St. Martin's Press

2   4   6   8   10   9   7   5   3   1   hardcover

Visit us on the Web at www.rodalestore.com, or call us toll-free at (800) 848-4735.

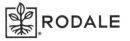

**WE INSPIRE AND ENABLE PEOPLE TO IMPROVE
THEIR LIVES AND THE WORLD AROUND THEM**

Natural Hormone Solutions Staff

EDITOR: Debra L. Gordon

WRITERS: Elizabeth Shimer, Marie Elaina Suszynski

CONTRIBUTING WRITERS: Jennifer Bright, Bridget Doherty, Patricia Dooley, Diane Kozak, Jennifer S. Kushnier, Elizabeth B. Price, Bebe Raupe, Alison Rice, Liz Sutherland, Mariska van Aalst, Julia VanTine

SERIES DESIGNER: Lynn N. Gano

COVER DESIGNER: Leanne Coppola

PHOTO EDITOR: Robin Hepler

ILLUSTRATORS: Shawn Banner, Judy Newhouse, Tom Ward

ASSISTANT RESEARCH MANAGERS: Sandra Salera Lloyd, Shea Zukowski

PRIMARY RESEARCH EDITOR: Anita C. Small

RESEARCH EDITORS: Carol J. Gilmore, Deborah Pedron

EDITORIAL RESEARCHERS: Molly Donaldson Brown, Jennifer Goldsmith, Karen Jacob, Jennifer S. Kushnier, Mary S. Mesaros, Elizabeth B. Price, Lucille Uhlman, Dorothy West, Teresa A. Yeykal

COPY EDITORS: Jean Rogers, Jane Sherman

EDITORIAL PRODUCTION MANAGER: Marilyn Hauptly

LAYOUT DESIGNER: Donna G. Rossi

MANUFACTURING COORDINATORS: Brenda Miller, Jodi Schaffer, Patrick T. Smith

Rodale Women's Health Books

EDITOR-IN-CHIEF: Tammerly Booth

VICE PRESIDENT OF MARKETING: Karen Arbegast

PRODUCT MARKETING DIRECTOR: Guy Maake

PRODUCT MANAGER: Dan Shields

MANUFACTURING MANAGER: Eileen Bauder

WRITING DIRECTOR: Jack Croft

RESEARCH DIRECTOR: Ann Gossy Yermish

MANAGING EDITOR: Madeleine Adams

ART DIRECTOR: Darlene Schneck

CONTENT ASSEMBLY MANAGER: Robert V. Anderson Jr.

DIGITAL PROCESSING GROUP MANAGERS: Leslie M. Keefe, Thomas P. Aczel

OFFICE STAFF: Julie Kehs Minnix, Catherine E. Strouse

Prevention Health Books for Women Board of Advisors

Contents

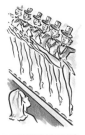
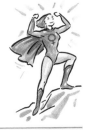

Introduction:
Don't Blame It on Hormones

How many times have you lashed out at your husband, burst into tears over a run in your stockings, or secretly gobbled the Häagen-Dazs by the light of the refrigerator and then blamed it on hormones?

Okay, so I'm describing my life. But I'm sure you can relate. We have this tendency to think that our hormones control us, particularly during *that* time of the month or during the months or years leading up to menopause. The truth is, while our hormones govern and direct nearly every function in our bodies, from our internal temperatures to our sexual desires to our hunger signals, they don't have to be the ones in control.

And that's the message of *Natural Hormone Solutions*. Whether you're just starting a new relationship with a wonderful man, trying to get pregnant, teaching your daughter about puberty, coping with the effects of aging, or simply looking for a way to avoid the monthly doldrums, this book will give you the tools you need. And we mean *tools*, not drugs—although medication is, of course, always an option in treating hormonal problems. But *Natural Hormone Solutions* reveals numerous natural ways—lifestyle and nutritional changes, exercises, herbs, supplements—to enhance the role of your hormones where necessary, tone down their actions where warranted, and protect you from the long-term damage some can wreak.

And while this isn't a book about menopause per se, we do devote two chapters to menopause. One describes the beauty and wonder inherent in this life change and shows how you can embrace and honor this passage. The other outlines the multitude of natural alternatives to hormone replacement therapy (HRT). But if you decide to go with HRT, we help you work through the pros and cons of treatment point by point, to make the best decision for *you*.

As in the other books in the Women's Edge health series, the advice in *Natural Hormone Solutions* is practical and doable. Most important, you'll learn that you can work with, not against, your natural hormone rhythms to improve virtually every aspect of your health.

Debra L. Gordon

Debra L. Gordon
Editor
Women's Edge Health Enhancement Guides

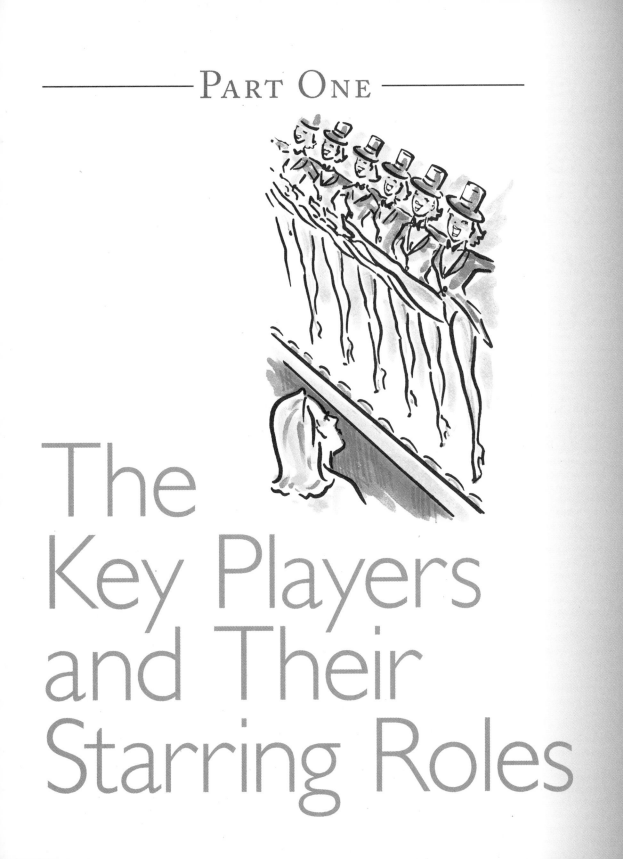

PART ONE

The Key Players and Their Starring Roles

Hormones: Pervasive, Powerful, and Profuse

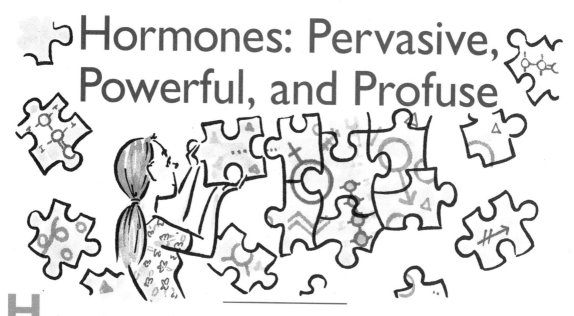

Here's a word guaranteed to get your mind going. *Hormones.*

Did you immediately think "periods"? "Menopause"? "Raging"? "Out of control"?

Or did the words *love, sex, weight loss,* and *calm* pop into your mind?

Think the latter images have nothing to do with the H-word? Think again.

Hormones influence who we are and nearly everything we do. When we go to sleep and when we wake up. Whether we're hungry or full. If we'll gain weight around our hips or our abdomens. Whether we want to have sex with our partners or simply cuddle our babies. Whether we're so depressed we can't get out of bed or so exuberant we're literally skipping down the street. They even determine how coordinated we are on any given day.

What hormones *don't* do is control us. So if we're gaining too much weight because we're not processing the hormone insulin properly, we can control it by exercising and changing our diets. "If your blood pressure is skyrocketing because your glands are pumping out too many stress hormones, you can change your lifestyle, learn some relaxation techniques, and bring those levels down," says Barbara Bartlik, M.D., assistant professor of psychology at the Weill Medical College of Cornell University in New York City. Even during the hormonal mania of menopause, when we blame nearly everything except the color of our eyes on our hormones, there are specific things we can do to pull the whole shebang back into balance.

But before you can begin controlling your hormones, you first have to understand the incredibly complex role they play in your body.

What Are Hormones, Anyway?

Think of the endocrine system as the postal service of the body. The letters are hormones, sent out by one of nine major glands and organs in the body. They're carried by the bloodstream, arriving at the correct postal box on certain cells, where, once opened and read, they deliver a set of specific instructions as to how that cell (and thus that body part) should behave. As with the postal service, the process can take seconds, as in response to a perceived threat, or it can occur over long stretches of time, as in providing the hormonal information that tells the body when and how to grow.

Overseeing the entire process is the hypothalamus, often called the master gland for its prominent role as a conductor in the orchestra of the endocrine system. It produces nine different hormones, called releasing hormones, that in turn trigger almost all the other glands in our bodies to turn either off or on.

Although a hormone travels throughout the body, it doesn't have an indiscriminate effect everywhere. Just like a letter is sorted by zip code, hormones are sorted by target cells. Then the actual street address—called a receptor site—is located on the target cells. Only the hormone with the same address as the receptor site fits. However, the same cell can have receptor sites for many different hormones. For example, the cells of the breast, uterus, and bones contain binding sites for estrogen, progesterone, testosterone, cortisol, and vitamin D—which, contrary to its name, is a hormone.

Hormone Overload

Sometimes, there are too many hormones, which can happen if you're prescribed an inappropriate dose or type of hormone replacement therapy. Then your body tries to bring you into balance in various ingenious ways.

The body may, for example, decrease the number of receptor sites

HORMONES AND VICES

You start your morning with a cup of coffee and a cigarette. You end your day with a few glasses of wine. Maybe you know these things could affect your heart, lungs, and even skin, but did you know they could also affect your hormones?

Too much caffeine can affect your stress hormones in much the same way as a fight with your husband. It increases secretion of ACTH, which is the hormone that triggers the adrenal glands to produce cortisol, the so-called stress hormone. Thus, it can lead to insomnia, anxiety, and even depression.

It may be a good idea to restrict or avoid caffeine—even the small amount of caffeine in decaffeinated coffee—during times of stress, and it's probably a good idea to avoid it if you have certain health conditions, such as high blood pressure, that are worsened by stress.

Alcohol can also increase adrenal hormone secretion. You may think of alcohol as a relaxant, but studies show alcohol can increase anxiety and interrupt normal sleep patterns. Alcohol can also interfere with your body's ability to use glucose and may lead to low blood sugar, especially on an empty stomach, after exercise, or during treatment with insulin or diabetes medication. Long-term, heavy alcohol consumption can also affect your menstrual cycle, suppress ovulation, and even bring on early menopause.

Women who smoke cigarettes are more likely to have osteoporosis and earlier menopause as well as the various risks associated with cardiovascular health and lung disease. Cigarette smoking also seems to increase your chances of irregular menstrual cycles, suggesting some connection with estrogen and progesterone.

But don't just quit willy-nilly. One study found that women who gave up smoking during the first half of their menstrual cycle (days 1 to 14 following menstruation, when estrogen levels are highest) had a much easier time withdrawing from tobacco and nicotine than women who quit during the second half, or luteal phase (day 15 and on, when progesterone levels are highest). One explanation is that the low mood that may occur during this time of your cycle, combined with withdrawal, could make quitting more difficult.

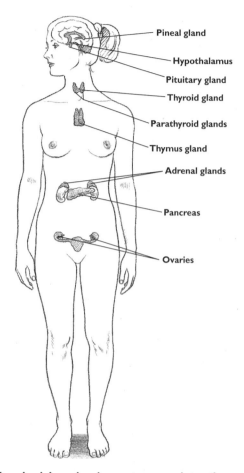

- Pineal gland
- Hypothalamus
- Pituitary gland
- Thyroid gland
- Parathyroid glands
- Thymus gland
- Adrenal glands
- Pancreas
- Ovaries

Your body's endocrine system regulates the complex network of hundreds of chemical messages we know as hormones. Here's a look at the major endocrine glands and organs in your body.

available or decrease the sensitivity of those receptor sites for that particular hormone. Kind of like hiding the mailbox behind a large tree. This is known as down-regulation.

Conversely, if you aren't getting enough of a particular hormone, your body tries to compensate by increasing the number and sensitivity of available receptor sites—or adding extra mailboxes. This is known as up-regulation.

Several complicated factors go into how well a target cell responds to a hormone; the hormone's concentration in the blood and the number of receptor sites are just two of them. Sometimes, a hormone's ability to work efficiently requires that another hormone be involved. So hormone A, for instance, primes the receptor sites to be ready for hormone B. Consider it hormonal foreplay.

For instance, an increase in estrogen leads not only to an increased number of receptor sites for estrogen but also to an increased number of receptor sites for the hormone progesterone. "This is probably because the two are interdependent," says Laurie Regan, N.D., Ph.D., a naturopathic physician in Portland, Oregon. That's why we have such a wide variety of symptoms—including breast tenderness, heavy menstrual flow, anxiety, or depression—when the two are out of balance, she says.

Dr. Regan also notes that often several hormones need to collaborate for physical events to happen. For example, the production of breast milk requires the collaborative effort of the hormones estrogen, progesterone, prolactin, and oxytocin.

Stimulating and Releasing Hormones

The hypothalamus secretes releasing hormones, such as TRH (thyroid releasing hormone), CRF (corticotropin releasing factor), and GnRH (gonadotropin releasing hormone), also known as LHRH (luteinizing hormone releasing hormone). These releasing hormones, in turn, trigger the pituitary gland to produce stimulating hormones, which include the various hormonal effects we're all familiar with.

Each hormone has specific triggers. For example, if you get too cold, a signal goes out to the hypothalamus to tell the thyroid to get going and produce more thyroid hormone. Your brain monitors the levels of thyroid hormone in the blood, and when the thyroid gland has produced enough to bring about the desired change (in this case, raising your core temperature), the information feeds back to the hypothalamus. The hypothalamus then turns off its production of TRH, signaling the pituitary gland to stop producing thyroid stimulating hormone, thus quelling the flow of thyroid hormone from the thyroid.

This feedback mechanism is how our bodies ensure we remain in a state of hormonal balance. But sometimes it seems like we have to work really hard to stay balanced. That's because many factors can influence our hormonal health, such as diet, stress, and illness.

Meet the Key Players

There are literally hundreds of hormones and hormone-like chemicals throughout your body. A chapter explaining them all would be longer than five of these books. But there are certain key players that make up the first string. They include:

DAVID AND GOLIATH: A BATTLE OF HORMONES?

It may well be that the duel between David and Goliath was the first known account of one opponent having a hormonally induced advantage over his rival. Only in this case, the advantage ironically came from a hormone imbalance and not from illegal supplementation. As it turned out, it was far from an advantage at all.

According to the biblical account, Goliath was about 10 feet tall. He was also slow-moving and had problems seeing the nimble David. These phenomena are consistent with the condition known as *acromegaly*. It's a disorder caused by too much growth hormone (often due to a tumor of the pituitary gland) that occurs once normal adult height is reached. Besides growing to gigantic proportions, someone with acromegaly might also have impaired eyesight, because the pituitary tumor can impinge on the optic nerve. That may explain why Goliath didn't see the stone coming at him.

It's not just the long bones of the skeleton that are affected by excessive secretion of growth hormone. The bones of the hands, feet, cheeks, and jaw thicken, and the eyelids, lips, tongue, and nose are also bigger. The jaw tends to protrude as a result of this thickening, and the cartilage around the vocal cords also increases, which can lead to a deep, husky voice, all features typically associated with giants in traditional fairy tales and biblical stories.

Acromegaly is a serious, debilitating condition. So it may be that the stone that struck Goliath's head and knocked him dead would have been the least of this Old Testament figure's problems.

The Stress Hormones

The car in front of you just slammed on its brakes, and you come to a screeching halt just inches from its bumper. You're breathing hard, your palms are damp, and your heart is pounding. The catecholamine hormones, epinephrine and norepinephrine, kick in within seconds to help you through the immediate alarm reaction. This is known as the sympathetic response. It's designed to help with the split-second decision of whether to fight back or get out of town, so your heart beats faster, your breathing rate increases, and your blood pressure rises. Then cortisol kicks in, helping you prepare for the longer haul of stress and recovery from some of its effects. It raises blood sugar levels to

BLAME IT ON HORMONES

Pharmaceutical Steroids

High doses of synthetic corticosteroid hormones like prednisone are often used to treat inflammatory conditions of the immune system such as asthma, Crohn's disease, and rheumatoid arthritis.

Studies suggest that in some instances, however, even short-term use of corticosteroids can suppress the natural ability of your adrenal glands to produce their own cortisol for several weeks, even after you stop taking the medication. During this time, your body's response to stress may still be impaired.

Additionally, one of the more common side effects of long-term corticosteroid use is osteoporosis. In just the first 3 to 6 months of using corticosteroids, you could see significant bone loss that's never fully regained, even when you stop taking the drugs.

In his newsletter, Andrew Weil, M.D., director of the integrative medicine program and clinical professor of internal medicine at the University of Arizona College of Medicine in Tucson, strongly recommends avoiding corticosteroid therapy wherever possible because of the devastating side effects from long-term use. He says corticosteroids suppress symptoms rather than addressing the underlying cause. Instead, he recommends an anti-inflammatory diet free of trans-fatty acids such as margarine and hydrogenated fats such as vegetable shortening. He advises including omega-3 fatty acids, found in flaxseed oil and fish such as salmon, mackerel, and trout.

It can be dangerous to abruptly stop taking your medications, however, so get your doctor's advice before making any changes to your therapy.

for your life. All reasons why chronic stress leads to greater susceptibility to infection, slow wound healing, and loss of sex drive.

In addition, prolonged cortisol secretion can increase levels of the hormone insulin. Among other things, insulin promotes fat storage, so chronic stress can actually make you gain weight and also make that weight harder to lose. You'll read more about the stress hormones in Fight or Flight: The Stress Hormones on page 52.

DHEA

Dehydroepiandrosterone, or DHEA, is a "hormone before a hormone," helping make testosterone and two of the three known types of estrogen: estrone and estradiol. In the body, DHEA can reverse some of the effects of excessive cortisol levels, thus helping reverse immune suppression and improve vitality.

"We maintain high levels until around the age of 25," says Dr. Regan. "After that, levels start to decline, which is why DHEA is associated with the idea of staying young."

But don't think of DHEA as any kind of fountain of youth. Many hormones decline as we age, and no one knows if supplementing with DHEA will keep us young. It's doubtful, though, because there are many more factors involved in aging than simply lower levels of DHEA. For more on this and other aging-re-

ensure you don't run out of fuel and helps divert energy away from those things—such as your immune and reproductive systems—that just don't matter quite so much when you're running

lated hormones, check out Staying Young: Aging and Hormones on page 71.

The Reproductive Hormones

More than any other hormones, it is estrogen and progesterone that truly make us women.

They work together in an interdependent cycle in which estrogen rises throughout the first half of the month to induce ovulation and then progesterone takes the lead, sending hormonal messages to build up the lining of the uterus for a baby. During pregnancy, when, of course, we're not ovulating, estrogen remains in the background, while progesterone dominates.

It's when the two are out of balance that we're left coping with such things as PMS, anxiety, breast tenderness, and uterine fibroids.

If you have problems ovulating, conceiving, or maintaining a pregnancy, chances are you have low levels of progesterone. Estrogen deficiencies can contribute to the development of osteoporosis and cardiovascular problems. For more on the role these two superstars play in reproduction, turn to Reproductive Health: Take Charge of Your Fertility on page 90.

Growth Hormone

Growth hormone does exactly what its name implies: enables our bodies to grow. Once we're all grown up, however, its role is to rebuild and repair our cells. "Growth hormone is highest at night when cortisol levels are supposed to be low, so our sleep can be restorative," says Dr. Regan. "If the opposite is happening due to stress overload, then the kinds of healing and repair that should occur when we're sleeping can't take place."

Growth hormone is another one that declines as we age, which is why some people think supplementing with it will postpone aging.

For more on growth hormone, see Staying Young: Aging and Hormones on page 71.

Insulin and Glucagon

Without insulin, we could eat all the food in the world and it would do us no good. Insulin is the passageway for food, which is transformed into glucose and absorbed by our cells to provide fuel for energy. Glucagon, the hormone that releases stored glucose, ensures there is enough glucose in the blood should levels fall below normal. This mechanism prevents low blood sugar levels at times when glucose is being used quickly, as when exercising, for example.

Major problems with insulin are characterized by either failure of our cells to respond to insulin (known as type 2, or adult-onset, diabetes) or an inability to produce insulin (type 1, or juvenile-onset, diabetes) so that our cells become deprived of fuel (glucose).

For more on insulin, see Insulin: When Sugar Ain't So Sweet on page 21.

Melatonin

Call this the "sleep hormone" because it plays an indispensable role in our sleep/wake cycles. Produced by the pineal gland, deep in the brain, melatonin should be highest at night, when it's dark, and lowest in the presence of light. We produce more melatonin during the winter than the summer (explaining that overwhelming urge to curl up under a soft blanket for mid-afternoon naps in January), so it has both a daily and a seasonal rhythm. It also interacts closely with the hormones that produce estrogen and progesterone, both of which are also involved in our ability to get a good night's sleep.

For more on melatonin, see Staying Young: Aging and Hormones on page 71.

Thyroxine and Triiodothyronine

Think of these hormones (collectively called thyroid hormone) as the superhormones of hormones. Thyroid hormones are masters at multitasking, crucial for maintaining our core temperatures and, therefore, our optimal metabolic rates. Translation: They determine how well we burn calories—ergo, how much of a problem we'll have with our weight. Thyroid hormones also regulate how our cells use oxygen and influence our growth and development.

Too much or too little of these valuable hormones throws off nearly every system in your body. Too little, called hypothyroidism, means you're dealing with everything from weight gain, sluggishness, depression, and constipation to the possibility of heart disease. Too much, called hyperthyroidism, may find you losing weight, missing sleep, nervous, and prone to diarrhea.

For more on the thyroid hormones, see The Thyroid: Energy for Everything on page 33.

Testosterone and Androstenedione

You may have thought of these as the sole property of your husband. But women also produce testosterone, although, thankfully, not in the same amounts as men. Primarily made in our ovaries and adrenal glands, it's nearly as important as candlelight and foreplay in terms of getting us in the mood for lovemaking.

ARE YOUR SEX HORMONES BALANCED?

Many of the symptoms attributed to sex hormone imbalances—such as irritability, anxiety, depression, lack of energy, joint pains, water retention, weight gain, and bloating—have their origins in digestive problems. For instance, blood sugar imbalance, food allergies, candidiasis (thrush or other infection caused by the yeastlike organism candida), and stress can all give rise to symptoms often associated with hormonal imbalances. Take the following quiz to determine the likelihood that your problem is caused by a hormone imbalance. If your answer to a question is yes, place a check mark in the box that follows. When you have answered all the questions, add up the number of boxes checked and record the total.

1. Do you use birth control pills? ❑
2. Do you ever experience joint pain? ❑
3. Do you experience water retention on a cyclical basis? ❑
4. Do you suffer from headaches on a cyclical basis? ❑
5. Do you have excess hair on your body or thinning hair on your scalp? ❑
6. Have you gained weight on your thighs and hips? ❑
7. Do you often suffer from mood swings? ❑
8. Are your mood swings cyclical? ❑
9. Do you suffer from fatigue or drowsiness during the day? ❑
10. Do you suffer from insomnia? ❑
11. Do you easily become irritable? ❑

Another sex-related, or androgenic, hormone is androstenedione. Yup, this is the same stuff St. Louis Cardinals hitter Mark McGwire took when he hit his record-breaking 62nd home run.

We usually convert androstenedione to estrogen in our fat cells. Sustained stress—such as severe dieting or starvation, which deplete our

12. Do you suffer from memory loss or poor concentration? ❑
13. Do you suffer from depression? ❑
14. Is your depression cyclical? ❑
15. Do you suffer from flatulence or bloating? ❑
16. Do you especially crave foods premenstrually? ❑
17. Have you at any time been bothered with problems affecting your reproductive organs? ❑
18. Do you have trouble conceiving or a history of miscarriage? ❑
19. Do you suffer from breast tenderness? ❑
20. Do you experience cramps or other menstrual irregularities? ❑
21. Are your periods often irregular or heavy? ❑
22. Do you suffer from lumpy breasts? ❑
23. Do you suffer from reduced libido? ❑
24. Do you often suffer from thrush? ❑
25. Do you suffer from constipation? ❑

Total: _____

Scoring

0–5: It is unlikely that you have a major hormonal imbalance.

6–14: There is a possibility that you have a degree of hormonal imbalance.

15–25: There is a strong probability that you have a sex hormone imbalance. Seek the guidance of a doctor, naturopath, or nutrition consultant, who can advise you about the need to test for hormone imbalances and tell you how to correct any.

fat stores—impairs our ability to convert it to estrogen. This can lead to a buildup of androgens and result in problems with estrogen and progesterone.

For more information on testosterone and other androgenic hormones, check out Testosterone: It's Not Just Your Husband's Hormone on page 42.

Hormones and Balance

If you think of balancing hormones at all, you probably think in terms of taking extra hormones, like estrogen during menopause. But that's only part of the story—a small part.

Hormonal balance is a critical component of *total* balance for optimal health and well-being. If you're addressing only one or two hormones or not thinking about them at all, then, yes, it's possible to become a slave to your hormones.

But that doesn't have to—and shouldn't—happen.

"I tell women that health and disease prevention are like a two-layered iced cake," says Susan Green Cooksey, Ph.D., a nurse practitioner and women's health care specialist at the Kaiser Center for Health Research in Portland, Oregon. "The two layers of the cake are all of the wellness behaviors and habits that we should put into practice. For example, exercising; eating a low-fat, high-fiber diet; controlling our weight and stress levels; not smoking; moderating caffeine and alcohol intake; and so on.

"Hormone replacement therapy, for instance, is merely the icing on the cake of wellness. It alone does little to prevent disease without a solid two-layer cake of wellness as its basis."

"From a holistic point of view, the same things that contribute to poor health in general can also trigger or exacerbate the symptoms of hormone imbalance," says Liz Sutherland, N.D., a naturopathic physician with the Natural Health Sciences Research Clinic in Lake Oswego, Oregon. "It's extremely important that women take the positive steps necessary to in-

SALIVA TESTS VERSUS BLOOD TESTS

Someday, getting an accurate measurement of your hormones may be as simple as spitting into a cup.

Already performed in some medical offices, testing saliva instead of blood for hormone levels offers several advantages.

- It's noninvasive, and you can do it in your home (you can order a kit and mail in the sample to a lab).
- You can collect several specimens at specified times. This is important because many hormones vary throughout the day. The ratio of morning to evening levels is as important to good health as the absolute levels.
- It may yield more accurate information in some instances because salivary hormone levels reflect the free or active hormone. Steroid hormones (estrogens, progesterone, testosterone, DHEA, and cortisol) are carried in the blood, attached to other molecules. When a hormone is bound this way, it is, in effect, unavailable for use. Measuring these hormone levels in the blood may be misleading because you don't know if the numbers reflect bound hormones or free and active hormone levels.

The main drawback to salivary hormone testing is that it's still relatively rare, and most medical personnel have little experience interpreting results. Salivary samples are not sterile, so if they are to be kept more than a week, they need to be frozen or have a preservative added. However, stability studies have shown that steroids are stable for the 5 to 7 days needed for proper shipping.

You can order a kit from any lab that does saliva testing. You don't have to do it through a doctor, although you will probably need a health care provider familiar with saliva testing to interpret the results. You collect the saliva yourself and mail it to the lab. Prices for both saliva and blood testing vary. Generally, saliva tests aren't covered by insurance.

Expert consulted
Lindsay Hofman, Ph.D.
Clinical chemistry consultant
Saliva Testing and Reference Laboratory
Vashon, Washington

form themselves about natural, effective, and safe options and why they would want to include those options in their wellness program, along with or, in some cases, instead of conventional medicines."

But it's important to be flexible, she says. "What helps balance the hormonal system of one woman may be different from what another woman needs."

Some natural options that Dr. Sutherland recommends include:

- Increasing your intake of phytoestrogens, natural plant hormones found in soy products, some fruits, and vegetables
- Eating organic animal products as much as possible, because they don't have extra hormones added to them
- Discussing with your doctor the use of natural hormone therapies such as bioestrogen and natural progesterone
- Taking a multivitamin/mineral and B complex to help counteract some effects of stress
- Using the herbs stinging nettle (*Urtica dioica*) and motherwort (*Leonurus cardiaca*) to optimize adrenal function and reduce the ill effects of stress on your body (see Fight or Flight: The Stress Hormones on page 52 for more information on stress)

In the following chapters, you'll find all of these suggestions—and more—spelled out clearly and simply, so that you, and you alone, can be the one in control of your hormones and, thus, of your body.

Estrogen: Friend or Foe?

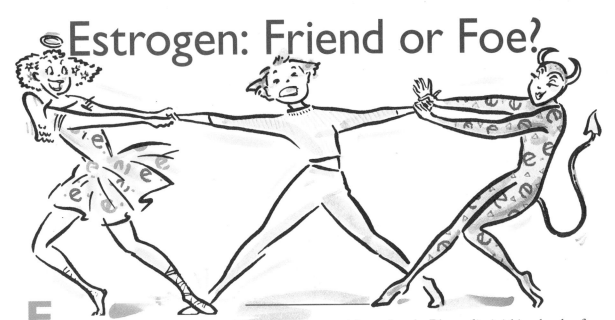

Estrogen is not just the little hormone waiting on the sidelines for its time of the month. Take it away, and we'd have to forfeit the game.

Estrogen lies at the very heart of our womanhood. Even though men have a bit of estrogen, it's not critical to their overall well-being.

Without it, though, our sex lives would be drier than the Sahara. Our skin as thin and brittle as crêpes. We'd be even more forgetful than we already are and would find *our* hairlines receding as fast as our husbands'. The difficulty isn't in naming the things estrogen *does* affect in our bodies; it's coming up with things estrogen *doesn't* affect.

Nearly all of estrogen's countless roles in our bodies are beneficial. And thankfully, even without taking supplemental estrogen in the form of hormone replacement therapy (HRT), there are many things we can do to help it along in its mission.

Estrogen and Skin: Teammates

Ahhh for the days when our faces looked taut all the time—not just when we pulled the skin up with our hands. Blame diminishing levels of estrogen for our "slowly sliding southward" skin. Of course, teenage days in the sun slathered with baby oil, coupled with vices like smoking and drinking also contribute, but in the first 5 years of menopause, we lose about 30 percent of our collagen, a protein that gives skin its plumpness and elasticity. Also, the fat layer under the skin that keeps it firm and resilient by stimulating the production of hyaluronic acid (which holds onto water like a camel to keep tissues moisturized) diminishes. The fact that these changes occur *after* menopause suggests they're related to estrogen loss, says Lila Nachtigall, M.D., professor of obstetrics and gynecology at New York University School of Medicine in New York City.

So in addition to the $50-an-ounce creams, we turn to face-lifts, laser peels (where the top layer of skin is removed), laser surgery (which zaps out wrinkles and spots), and Botox (botulinum toxin type A), in which actual poison is injected into the face to paralyze the muscles we use to frown and smile.

One touted benefit of estrogen replacement

ESTROGEN: AS UNIQUE AS A WOMAN

Like moods and menstrual cycles, estrogen levels vary in percentage and presence over the course of your lifetime. So far, researchers have identified three main types of estrogen—estradiol, estrone, and estriol—although they think there may be more.

Often termed the *natural estrogen*, estradiol is the strongest form and is made by the ovaries during normal menstrual cycles. Estriol is the weakest form; it's called the pregnancy estrogen and is formed by the placenta. Estrone is somewhere in the middle in terms of strength. It's the estrogen of menopause, formed in fat and muscle.

We all have different levels and ratios of the three types in our systems, depending on genetic background and stage in life. And these levels can mean different things for our health. For example, Asian women naturally have more estriol than Caucasian women, as do women who have had early pregnancies. These high estriol levels may partially block some of the effects of the more-potent estrogen forms, thereby decreasing the risk of certain conditions (such as breast cancer) linked to potent estrogen.

therapy (ERT) is that it can prevent up to one-third of the collagen loss we experience in those first years after menopause and help to maintain the fat layer beneath the skin. But once skin has improved to a certain point, taking estrogen long term doesn't appear to make any difference.

However, if you hit menopause with healthy skin, the damage that does occur won't seem quite as major. Even without HRT, there are some postmenopause things you can do to strengthen your skin.

Oil your insides. To keep your skin soft and supple, you must first get enough essential fatty acids internally, particularly the omega-3 fatty acids, says Ellen Kamhi, R.N., Ph.D., author of *Cycles of Life: Herbs and Energy Techniques for Women.* "These are found in flaxseed oil and cer-tain fish, including tuna, salmon, and herring," she says. Just two to three servings a week of fish rich in omega-3s is enough to keep laugh lines at bay. Enhance the effect by taking 1 tablespoon of flaxseed oil a day for every 100 pounds of body weight.

Put on a sesame suit. You need to lube up on the outside, too. "Ancient Ayurvedic medicine suggests you put a thin layer of sesame oil all over your entire body and let it soak in for a few minutes before you get into the shower," says Dr. Kamhi. (To prevent slipping, don't oil up your feet, though.) Sesame oil works well because it is easily absorbed, and what's left washes off quickly without leaving a residue. It works especially well when it is mixed with a few drops of vitamin E, she says. Just break open a vitamin E capsule and add it to the sesame oil. Premix a couple of ounces of this and store it in a dark plastic bottle in your shower.

Do some chin-ups. Facial exercises oxygenate the skin and make it more elastic, says Dr. Kamhi. Here's one good exercise for under the chin: Put the top of your hand against the bottom of your chin and push up. With the muscles at the bottom of your face, press down on the top of your hand. Hold for 10 seconds and release. Repeat this exercise 10 times twice daily. "Don't worry about making a funny face—this exercise will tighten everything under your chin," she says.

Estrogen and Depression: Rivals

"Estrogen makes women feel good," says Martha Louise Elks, M.D., professor of medicine at the Morehouse School of Medicine in Atlanta. It seems to raise levels of the feel-good hormone, serotonin, making us more mellow and flexible in how we react to whatever life throws us. "We still notice life's injustices, but we're not so bothered by them," Dr. Elks says. "We say, 'Yeah, he's a jerk—men are jerks. So what?'"

Try that philosophy the week before your period, or just after you've given birth, when your estrogen levels are low. Then your response is likely to be, "Yeah, he's a jerk," as you slam the door/throw the plate/storm out of the room. Studies show depression and even suicide attempts are more frequent during estrogen lulls. "There's a mistaken impression that when a woman is having her period, she's a bitch," says Dr. Elks. "But actually, it's during her flow that a woman's estrogen levels are rising, and she's feeling better."

Conventional treatments for depression include a variety of antidepressant drugs, psychotherapy, and a combination of both. According to a study reviewing medical literature on women and depression published in the *Journal of the American Menopause Society*, estrogen replacement therapy also seems to help women with peri- and postmenopausal depression.

While you should seek help from a qualified mental health expert for any sign of depression, there are also proven natural alternatives for mild-to-moderate depression to keep in mind. Try these.

Illuminate yourself. "Before we use any herbs or supplements, we need to find out what's causing the depression," says Dr. Kamhi. Sometimes it's something relatively simple, like lack of sunlight, which can be treated with a light box. Light treatment should be considered even before using herbs, she says, because there are no chemicals or toxicities in light, and you can op-

erate a light box at work or at home. Use this treatment only in consultation with your doctor, who can explain proper use of the box and set up an appropriate treatment schedule.

Brew a soothing tea. "My favorite antidepressant is a tea made of Siberian ginseng and rosebuds—it immediately lifts your spirits," says Dr. Kamhi. Get Siberian ginseng from a health food store in the form of the whole root, in a tea bag, or in a capsule.

Try some other spirited remedies. Consider SAM-e (S-adenosylmethionine), a nutritional supplement that has been used for years in Europe to treat depression and has more recently been introduced into the United States. Take 600 to 1,200 milligrams daily. St. John's wort is also excellent, says Dr. Kamhi. Kava kava is a good antianxiety herb, she says. Follow label directions for dosage.

Move for your mood. Physical activity is a great way to prevent and treat depression. Researchers don't know exactly why exercise helps, but they suggest it may enhance our sense of mastery, so we feel more mentally and physically in control. Aerobic activity may also help vent pent-up frustration. And mood-enhancing beta-endorphins (responsible for the runner's high) released during exercise could also be involved. Aim for at least 30 minutes of exercise most days. If you want, you can break it into three sets of 10 minutes each.

Expand your exercise horizons. Yoga and tai chi are excellent depression remedies. For one thing, if you take a class, you'll bond with others, says Dr. Kamhi. Also, some movements and breathing exercises in yoga and tai chi can stimulate glands to release mood-enhancing hormones. For example, the shoulder stand in yoga increases circulation to the thyroid gland.

Grab your partner. A study published in the *Journal of Nervous and Mental Disease* found that a supportive spouse and other positive relationships reduced the likelihood of major depression.

Estrogen and the Brain: Allies

You finish putting the groceries into the trunk and slam the lid down just as you realize your keys are next to the dog food. Or you run through a litany of names before hitting on your 12-year-old's actual moniker. And most mornings, you wind up lathering twice when you wash your hair because you can't remember if you already used shampoo. Could it be your estrogen is a bit on the low side?

Thank estrogen for keeping you tops in the mental game. It seems to work by protecting nerve cells in the brain. Picture your brain cells as the branches on a tree. Each of those branches, called dendritic spines, has its own smaller twigs, called dendrites, which reach out to other twigs to pass information. As you gain years, you naturally lose dendrites, which leads to fading memory. Estrogen helps preserve dendrites and dendritic spines, protecting your memory.

Estrogen also plays a role in the manufacture of the memory-preserving neurotransmitter acetylcholine, which also tends to decline with age. Researchers speculate that estrogen drops may be related in some way to Alzheimer's disease (AD), which is connected with acetylcholine drops. "As far as Alzheimer's disease is concerned, it's unknown whether or not estrogen can actually delay or prevent it," says Rachelle Doody, M.D., Effie Marie Cain professor in Alzheimer's disease research at Baylor College of Medicine in Houston. But there are some theories.

Besides the decline in acetylcholine in Alzheimer's disease, there's a death of neurons (nerve cells), especially in the learning and memory areas of the brain. This nerve cell death is triggered both by a buildup of protein deposits called B-amyloid and by abnormal tangles in the neuron fibers. Estrogen is thought to curb the effects of B-amyloid buildup in the brain by decreasing the amount of apolipoprotein B (a chemical that magnifies the effects of the B-amyloid deposits).

Estrogen also increases blood flow to the arteries in our necks, which helps more blood get to our brains. And increased blood helps keep our brain cells healthy and enables them to use blood sugar for energy. Likewise, estrogen reduces the amount of chemicals in our brains that cause inflammation—another problem associated with AD.

Interestingly, more thin than obese women get Alzheimer's disease, perhaps because estrogen is stored in fat, further evidence that suggests estrogen may help fight AD. Conventionally, there are drugs that slow the progression of AD, as well as medications that treat the depression that often accompanies it.

Estrogen replacement therapy is also an option. It seems to stall the deterioration of the short- and long-term memory loss that occurs with normal aging and with Alzheimer's disease. And, according to some very preliminary research, women already suffering from the early stages of AD who take estrogen may show fewer signs of the disease than those who don't take it.

But the best approach to memory loss and Alzheimer's disease is prevention and mental fitness, says Maria Sulindro, M.D., president and founder of eAntiAging.com, an Internet organization that provides scientific information about antiaging approaches. "Once someone has it, it's not so easy to reverse," she says. She and other experts suggest the following.

Give your brain a workout. "Your brain is just like the muscles in your body—if you don't use it, you lose it," says Dr. Kamhi. Thinking about things that are a stretch, like a 14-step calculus problem or how to say "I'm hungry for pizza" in a foreign language, can increase nerve transmission in your brain, preserving your memory.

Hang upside down. Yoga—especially the inverted positions—is particularly good for the brain, says Dr. Kamhi. "Using a slant board can help get more blood and nutrients to your brain." To make one, prop one end of a plank of wood or an ironing board against a chair. Be sure that it is secured properly and can hold your weight. Then lie on it with your feet at the upper end and your head at the lower end. "Check with your doctor. If she feels this is appropriate for you, do this three times a week for 20 to 30 minutes," says Dr. Kamhi. When the exercise ends, get back on your feet slowly and carefully.

Try some supplements and herbs. "Vitamin C is thought of as one of the common vitamins that can improve brain and mental functions," says Dr. Sulindro. Take 1,000 to 2,000 milligrams of vitamin C (ascorbyl palmitate) daily. L-tyrosine and other amino acids can also help. Take 200 milligrams of tyrosine and 1,000 to 2,000 milligrams of L-glutamine daily.

Dr. Kamhi suggests working with your doctor and a qualified alternative practitioner to see if the following herbs are right for you.

> ❧ *Periwinkle.* It increases circulation to the brain. Take 1,000 milligrams of *Vinca minor* a day as a liquid extract.

WHAT ARE SERMs?

They're "selective estrogen receptor modulators," and they imitate the action of estrogen. They latch on to spots in the body where their estrogen-like actions do good, while avoiding areas where they're likely to cause harm. For example, a SERM might fight against cardiovascular disease—without the potentially cancer-causing effects of estrogen in the uterus. It's sort of like the body is a party, and upon arrival, the SERMs bypass their enemies and meet up with their friends.

Some experts have termed SERMs "designer estrogens." It's not fully known exactly how they work. Theories suggest that an individual SERM stimulates only certain estrogen receptors, so it interacts only with the tissues it affects in a good way, not with tissues that it may affect negatively.

The first widely used SERM was tamoxifen citrate, a drug derived from yew trees that has been used since 1978 as a treatment for breast cancer and a means to increase bone density. A 1998 study published in the *Journal of the National Cancer Institute* suggested that tamoxifen may also be effective for breast cancer *prevention*. This use is somewhat controversial, however, because a report on a 1999 study in the same journal revealed that tamoxifen may increase the risk of endometrial cancer.

Raloxifene (Evista) is another SERM. This drug mimics estrogen's positive effects on bone density and blood lipids. At the same time, it lowers the risk of breast cancer and may lower the risk of uterine cancer.

There are also natural SERMs: phytoestrogens. They're compounds found in some plants we eat, such as soybeans and flaxseed. A study published in the *European Journal of Obstetrics and Gynecology* suggests that phytoestrogens may help prevent heart disease and osteoporosis, without the increased breast cancer risk that comes with estrogen.

> ❧ *Ginkgo biloba.* This well-researched herb has been shown to increase circulation to the brain. Take 240 milligrams each morning as a capsule or liquid extract.

- *Phosphatidylserine.* This is a fatty substance in brain cells that decreases with age. Studies show that amounts increase in the brain when phosphatidylserine is taken orally. It's also known to increase brain electrical activity. Take a 300-milligram capsule once a day.
- *Acetyl-L-carnitine.* Tested specifically on Alzheimer's disease patients, this amino acid may help the brain use fat correctly, which could help lessen the development of plaques seen in the disease. Take 150 milligrams a day as a capsule.
- *Huperzine A (HupA).* A Chinese remedy made from club moss, HupA appears to stop the breakdown of the brain enzyme acetylcholinesterase. A study conducted at the Chinese Academy of Sciences suggests that HupA may be a good therapy to treat or prevent Alzheimer's disease.

BLAME IT ON HORMONES
Hair Loss

Sure, men fret when they go bald. Some grow their remaining hair longer in the front or on one side and then comb it to cover their bare domes. Some even get a toupee. But no matter how they cope, they have millions of other men with whom to share their pain.

Baldness is different in women. We're not *supposed* to go bald. "And with all the work that's gone into male pattern baldness, the issue in women has been relatively ignored," says Ellen W. Seely, M.D., director of clinical research in the endocrine-hypertension division at Brigham and Women's Hospital in Boston.

Most balding in women is caused by a condition known as androgenic alopecia (AGA)—the same condition that causes the majority of male baldness. You can blame your genes if you have it. "Many women with this problem had grandmothers who had it, and great-grandmothers who had it," says Dr. Seely.

But you can also blame your hormones. Testosterone, for one. Too much (in men or women) means you're more likely to lose the hair on your head yet *grow* hair on other parts of

Estrogen and the Heart: Comrades

"We know that being premenopausal is protective against heart disease," says Ellen W. Seely, M.D., director of clinical research in the endocrine-hypertension division at Brigham and Women's Hospital in Boston. "Estradiol (the estrogen made by the ovaries) is present in premenopausal women but falls to very low levels with menopause," says Dr. Seely. Estrogen increases HDL (good) cholesterol, lowers LDL (bad) cholesterol, improves blood vessel dilation, and may reduce cholesterol buildup in the aorta. All of these actions may ward off heart disease.

Estrogen also helps relax the muscles around the blood vessels, so they don't squeeze and narrow at the wrong time. Estrogen may also help prevent blood clots in premenopausal women.

It seems logical, therefore, to believe that giving estrogen to women *after* menopause would help protect them. However, estrogen replacement therapy (ERT), as it is currently prescribed, has *not* passed the test as a preventative method against heart disease. Although many observational studies suggest ERT helps protect against heart disease, the HERS study published in the *Journal of the American Medical Association* found that postmenopausal women with a his-your body. A woman with this problem will go bald in the same places as her husband: on her temples and the top of her head, while growing hair on her chin, under her belly button, and on her inner thighs and lower back. This kind of unusual hair growth or loss could also indicate a medical problem other than AGA, so it should be checked out by an endocrinologist, says Dr. Seely.

Estrogen, on the other hand, has the opposite effect on scalp hair in that it *prolongs* the length of the hair follicle. "So with more estrogen, the hair can grow longer, and there's more hair on the scalp," says Dr. Seely. This explains why women experience some hair loss after childbirth and menopause, when estrogen levels fall. It also explains why we can grow our hair longer than most men.

If you're concerned about baldness, first make sure there isn't a medical issue. "Tumors can make male hormone, which can cause baldness," Dr. Seely says. Apart from that, hair is dependent on diet and stress level. "So avoiding major stresses and getting enough vitamins can help," she says. Other treatments that have been reported to work in some studies include exotic herbs, amino acids, and a soft laser scalp massage. Drugs for balding include topical minoxidil (Loniten) and the pill finasteride (Proscar).

Chill out. Researchers aren't quite sure exactly how stress affects our hearts, but they do know that stress increases levels of cortisol, which in turn accelerates the aging process. The aging process has a connection to heart disease, which is one of the most common age-related diseases and the leading cause of death in postmenopausal women. Also, when we're stressed, we tend to turn to heart-harming practices like drinking, smoking, or overeating to help compensate.

For numerous stress-reducing remedies, see Fight or Flight: The Stress Hormones on page 52.

Take fat-soluble vitamin C (ascorbyl palmitate). Vitamin C keeps the arterial walls from thinning as we age, says Dr. Sulindro. When the walls thin, they have a tendency to crack and leak. This process causes inflammation, enabling the undesirable LDL cholesterol to accumulate along the inner walls of the coronary arteries. The most common form of vitamin C, ascorbic acid, is water soluble and won't reach the vascular wall, says Dr. Sulindro. "Instead, take 1,000 to 2,000 milligrams of fat-soluble vitamin C, ascorbyl palmitate. This form stays in the body longer, having more chance to get to the arterial wall," she says.

Ask about amino acids. L-lysine and L-proline can help clear the LDL cholesterol that clogs blood circulation. "This clogging represents half of all deaths of heart disease patients," says Dr. Sulindro. Get your doctor's approval before taking these amino acids. For stroke prevention, folic acid also seems to work. Take 800 micrograms daily.

Make it beat. Couch potato syndrome can raise your heart disease risk to match that of a

tory of heart disease who took estrogen didn't lower their risk of a heart attack.

Other research suggests that taking estrogen orally may increase the chance of leg blood clots for postmenopausal women during the first year of use. "ERT as used in the HERS study is not the same as the natural estrogen women have circulating in their bodies prior to menopause," says Dr. Seely. "So if we could give postmenopausal women estrogen more similar to the natural form they have before menopause, it might actually be protective."

For now, experts agree that the best protection against heart disease and stroke is prevention. Here are some good strategies.

pack-a-day smoker or a woman who is 20 percent overweight. So get at least 30 minutes of accumulated exercise a day at a pace equivalent to brisk walking.

Get fishy. Omega-3 fatty acids in fish appear to fight heart disease. An Italian study showed that over time, the death rate in a group of patients who had had heart attacks within the previous 3 months dropped 14 to 20 percent when they took fish-oil capsules. "Eat fresh fish three times a week or ask your doctor about using supplements," Dr. Sulindro says.

Estrogen and Sleep: A Love/Hate Relationship

You toss and turn, staring at the ceiling, counting more sheep than there are in England. Is it the big report due tomorrow? Braces for your teenager? The plummeting stock market? Could be. Then again, it could be your plummeting estrogen levels.

The sleep-controlling areas of the brain, the hypothalamus and the hippocampus, contain cells with certain parts made just for estrogen, called estrogen receptors. Like the proverbial lock and key, estrogen in the blood seeks out these receptors, glomming onto them and passing on their chemical messages. Scientists think that when this process occurs, estrogen helps with sleep by altering levels of other brain chemicals that play a part in our sleep patterns, like acetylcholine, dopamine, and serotonin. And because estrogen alleviates other discomforts, such as night sweats, vaginal dryness, and

REAL-LIFE SCENARIO
Her Doctor Wants Her to Have a Hysterectomy

Maeve, 52, has had fibroids most of her life. Since she's finished having children, her doctor now recommends a hysterectomy to get rid of the fibroids once and for all. But Maeve doesn't like the idea of removing her uterus, even if she is through with childbearing. What are her options?

Hysterectomies are way overdone in this country. If Maeve doesn't want to have a hysterectomy, she may not need to. First, she should get a clear reason from her physician as to *why* she needs the surgery and what the alternatives are. She should also seek a second opinion. Additionally, for a 52-year-old woman, menopause is at hand, and fibroids tend to shrink with menopause.

Some clear reasons to have a hysterectomy include cancer of the cervix, endometrial cancer, severe dysplasia (precancer) of the lining of the uterus, or a more rare condition of severe, life-threatening bleeding requiring transfusions. Yet another reason would be the presence of recurrent, more aggressive precancerous cells of the cervix. The precancerous changes may initially be treated locally by freezing or by "cone" surgery of the cervix. Only if these options are unsuccessful or if the precancer condition keeps returning should Maeve opt for the hysterectomy.

Fibroids are lumps of muscular tissue that grow in response to estrogen. During a woman's reproductive years, there are regular and cyclic estrogen increases that over time may cause these noncancerous growths. And fibroids may occur in inconvenient places. Myomectomy, removal of the fibroid alone, may be an option for Maeve. While size ("as large as an orange") has been regarded by some gyne-

some urinary conditions, it also indirectly helps us get much-needed rest. That's why we may have more problems sleeping just before our periods or when we're pre- or postmenopausal—those times are when estrogen levels drop.

cologists as the reason to remove the tumor, there is no evidence that failing to do so will shorten Maeve's life.

If Maeve is uncomfortable or bleeding heavily, she should first confirm that the fibroids are to blame. She may opt for hormonal management of her bleeding. This usually involves taking progesterone in the form of medroxyprogesterone. The oral forms are not the natural hormone, and Maeve, like some women, might have minor to moderate side effects—PMS-type feelings such as bloating, headaches, breast tenderness, and joint pain. Another approach Maeve and her doctor might consider to alleviate the heavy bleeding involves outpatient surgery called D and C (dilatation and curettage that removes the uterine lining).

Today, many women and their doctors falsely view the uterus as the cause of many female ills, and its removal becomes almost routine. True, if a woman is having heavy or annoying periods and doesn't tolerate the medication to help alleviate this, a hysterectomy would be the solution.

But Maeve should be aware that the usual surgery—total hysterectomy with removal of the tubes and ovaries—may result in her using estrogen longer than women who never had the surgery. There are both risks and benefits to prolonged postmenopausal estrogen use.

These are all issues that should not be decided by a woman alone. She needs the advice of a knowledgeable and sympathetic physician. With persistence and effort, she should be able to find such an individual.

Expert consulted
Martha Louise Elks, M.D.
Professor of medicine
Morehouse School of Medicine
Atlanta

ment, high estrogen levels may put some romance into your dreamworld with sexual dreams strong enough to wake you up, says Dr. Elks.

Although there are a variety of other reasons for sleep problems and a plethora of prescription medications, including hormone replacement therapy, that may help you sleep, says Dr. Sulindro, there are also numerous alternative methods. Try these.

- *Kava kava (Piper methysticum).* It reduces anxiety, restlessness, and stress, all of which can disrupt sleep. Take 50 to 100 milligrams daily.
- *St. John's wort (Hypericum perforatum).* Primarily used as an antidepressant, St. John's wort can also reduce toss-and-turn anxiety. Take 50 to 100 milligrams daily.
- *Vitamin D.* It relaxes your mind and your muscles. You can get your daily dose from 15 minutes of daily sunlight, and you can also take it in supplement form. The suggested daily intake is 400 international units (IU), but Dr. Sulindro says you need only 100 to 300 IU in supplement form.

If you want to improve your sleep without downing any supplements, you have other options. The National Sleep Foundation recommends these approaches.

Don't nap. Napping during the day can affect your ability to fall asleep at night.

Get into a sleep routine. Regular, established bedtime rituals, like darkness or a hot bath, signal your brain that it's time for bed.

Estrogen also plays a role in our dreams. More amorous, sexual dreams typically occur at mid-cycle, when estrogen levels are high and we're at our most fertile. Makes sense. And if your sex life is about as exciting as a 401(k) state-

Abstain from coffee and beer. When consumed in the afternoon or evening, caffeine can keep you awake and alcohol can interrupt your sleep.

Make your bed a shrine to sleep. Use your bed only for sleeping (or sex), so you associate it with sleep.

Estrogen and Wounds: Buddies

When you are wounded, even if it's just a wince-worthy paper cut, estrogen plays a vital role in the healing process. Estrogen is chemically similar to a steroid, explains Manish Suthar, M.D., physician at the Texas Back Institute in Plano, and steroids are the basic fundamental products our cells use for growth, development, and maintenance.

Some ways to improve wound healing and (hopefully) speed estrogen's effects include:

Reach for buffered C. Vitamin C sparks healthy cell growth. "I recommend taking 1,000 milligrams of ascorbic acid powder buffered with calcium and magnesium," says Dr. Kamhi. This should be a substitute for any vitamin C supplement you are taking, rather than an addition to it, she adds.

Digest the wound. Put a small amount of powdered digestive enzymes, such as bromelain and papain, directly onto the wound. You can open a capsule or buy the enzymes in powdered form. "They help the cut heal, especially if it's open," Dr. Kamhi says.

Seal it. Once it starts to heal, pack the injury with aloe vera gel and goldenseal powder to speed up the process, says Dr. Kamhi. Mix 1 tablespoon of the gel with ½ teaspoon of goldenseal powder. The goldenseal acts as an antimicrobial so the cut doesn't get infected, and the aloe soothes it and may also increase blood flow, speeding healing. Once a seal has formed on the cut, dressing it with vitamin E may help decrease scarring. "You can open a vitamin E capsule and apply the contents, or you can use vitamin E oil," Dr. Kamhi says.

Insulin: When Sugar Ain't So Sweet

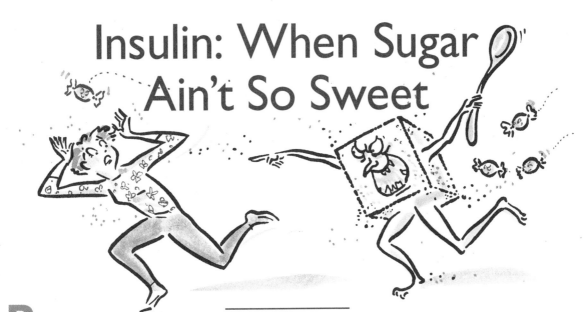

Blame it on overeating and underexercising: Type 2 diabetes, which is associated with obesity and a sedentary lifestyle, is reaching epidemic proportions—with women leading the pack.

Although just 6½ percent of the entire population has diabetes—a disease in which the body can't make enough of the hormone insulin or can't use insulin to convert food into energy—9 percent of women have it. And it's the seventh leading cause of death in this country.

Researchers estimate that by the year 2020, about 250 million people throughout the world may have impaired glucose tolerance, a condition in which their blood sugar is continuously too high, which puts them at significant risk for type 2 diabetes.

Those are grim numbers, but there's good news. While there are some risks for developing type 2 diabetes that we can't control, like genetic makeup and age, diabetes is also linked to two things we *can* control: weight and activity level. Healthy eating and exercising may help us not only dodge diabetes but also avoid complications if we do get the disease.

How a Hormone Can Go Wrong

When you eat, your food turns into glucose, or sugar, and heads out into your bloodstream looking for cells to latch onto, like a new divorcée in a singles bar. Enter insulin, a hormone that's released by beta cells in the pancreas when you eat. Insulin attaches to cell receptors all over your body, acting like a chaperone and determining if glucose can enter those cells to provide your muscles and other organs the energy they need.

But sometimes, the system goes wrong.

In type 1 diabetes, also called juvenile diabetes because it usually occurs in childhood, the immune system mistakenly attacks and kills beta cells, so your body can't make *any* insulin. The only treatment in this case involves daily injections of synthetic insulin to get glucose into your cells.

In type 2 diabetes, also called adult-onset diabetes because it usually occurs after age 45, the body doesn't properly use the insulin, so it's not able to usher the glucose into the cells. Doctors call this "insulin resistance." As a result, sugar ends up staying in your bloodstream instead of being converted to energy. This signals the pancreas to try to fix things, so it starts pumping out even *more* insulin, believing there's all this extra glucose to shepherd into cells. At this point, you're considered insulin resistant. You may not have any obvious symptoms, however, other than an inability to lose weight (and you're probably already overweight).

If the beta cells can't keep up with the increased demand for insulin, you develop full-fledged type 2 diabetes. Your food isn't turned into energy, and glucose is constantly circulating through your bloodstream, putting you at long-term risk for eye, kidney, nerve, and heart damage.

Recognize Your Risks

Women, in particular, need to work to prevent diabetes because we have more risks than men. For instance:

We live longer. We may age gracefully, but every year we live past 45 increases our risk of diabetes. And since women live longer than men, you can figure out the end result.

We're hippy. Women are more likely to be overweight than men are. And once we're 35 to 40 percent over our ideal body weight, we're 40 percent less sensitive to insulin.

We love (and need) our conveniences. Like men, we've fallen into a more sedentary lifestyle. We burn fewer calories to get around, to change the channel, even to do housework. But since so many women are working two shifts—a day at the office and then a night of cooking, dish washing, and laundry—we're more likely to use calorie-saving conveniences than men.

We bear the children. About 5 percent of pregnant women develop gestational diabetes, a form of type 2 diabetes, during their third trimester. Pregnancy tends to make women more insulin resistant, but those who develop gestational diabetes appear to have an inherent weakness in the beta cells, so they are unable to make enough insulin. The insulin resistance and blood sugar levels usually return to normal after delivery, but up to one-half of these women develop type 2 diabetes within 10 years after childbirth.

The risk of developing type 2 diabetes is even higher in women who've had gestational diabetes and who take the progestin-only birth control pill while breastfeeding, says Ruanne Peters, Sc.D., professor of preventive medicine at the University of Southern California in Los Angeles. That may be because progesterone, the natural form of the synthetic hormone progestin, tends to increase insulin resistance. Estrogen, which may counterbalance the effects of progestin, is low in women who are breastfeeding. And although other birth control pills contain estrogen, doctors usually don't prescribe them for women who are breastfeeding.

Beyond gender, there are other attributes that can increase your risk of developing type 2 diabetes, including:

Ethnicity. If you're a Latina, African-American, Asian, Pacific Islander, or Native American, you're more likely to develop diabetes. Latina women are almost twice as likely as Caucasian women to get the disease.

Growth hormone therapy in childhood. Growth hormone therapy increases production of insulin and thus insulin resistance, rendering children who took it six times more likely to develop type 2 diabetes as adults.

Use of prescription beta-blockers. Researchers at Johns Hopkins University found that people who *didn't* have diabetes when they started taking beta-blockers for high blood pressure and heart disease were 28 percent more likely to develop the disease than those who didn't take the medication. One reason is that beta-blockers have a huge impact on the method by which glucose is turned into energy. If you have several other risk factors for diabetes, talk to your doctor about using other medications, such as thiazide diuretics, ACE inhibitors, and calcium-channel antagonists, for your blood pressure and heart condition.

High cholesterol levels. High levels of "bad" LDL cholesterol, low levels of "good" HDL cholesterol, and high triglycerides (the amount of fat in the blood) are often found in people with type 2 diabetes. These conditions are also risk factors for heart disease. HDL cholesterol protects against heart disease, so when it's low but LDL cholesterol and triglycerides are high, the fats in your blood can cause blockages, resulting in angina, a heart attack, or sudden death.

Sum Up Your Symptoms

Half of the 16 million Americans who have diabetes don't even know they have it. That's why every woman over the age of 45 should be tested for diabetes every 3 years, whether or not she feels any symptoms, says Lynne M. Kirk, M.D., associate chief of the division of internal medicine at the University of Texas Southwestern Medical Center in Dallas.

WOMEN ASK WHY
What is Syndrome X?

Otherwise known as metabolic syndrome, Syndrome X consists of a cluster of heart disease risk factors, including obesity, high insulin levels, high blood pressure, and hyperlipidemia (elevated levels of fat in the blood). It is characterized by insulin resistance, which is when the body has a difficult time converting glucose into energy.

In those with Syndrome X, the pancreas pumps out large amounts of insulin, which gets only some of that glucose into cells. Diabetes doesn't usually occur, but glucose levels are usually at the upper end of the normal range.

The following factors put women with insulin resistance at higher risk for heart disease:

- High triglycerides (the amount of fat in the blood)
- Low HDL ("good") cholesterol levels
- High blood pressure
- Dense LDL ("bad") cholesterol particles (which can get into the arteries more easily and cause blockages)
- Accumulation of lipoproteins (which help triglycerides travel throughout the bloodstream)
- Lower ability to break up blood clots

Syndrome X is strongly associated with obesity. In fact, being overweight is one of its most common signs. Extra body fat lowers your sensitivity to insulin and puts you at increased risk of heart disease.

Treatment includes losing weight, even if it's only 10 or 15 pounds, and exercise. The exercise does more than help with the weight loss. It also increases insulin sensitivity and lowers blood pressure. If medication is needed, a doctor usually prescribes statins, which lower blood lipids.

Expert consulted
Lila A. Wallis, M.D., M.A.C.P.
Clinical professor of medicine
Weill Medical College of Cornell University
New York City

If you are in a high-risk group, your testing should start at a younger age, says Dr. Kirk. (Risks include having a family history of the disease, belonging to an at-risk ethnic group, and being overweight.)

Measuring the amount of sugar, or glucose, in your blood is the only way your doctor can know for sure if you have the disease. People with diabetes have above-normal blood sugar levels even if they haven't eaten in a while.

Normal blood sugars fall within a range of 70 to 120. Mild cases of diabetes usually fall in the low- to mid-100 range. Severe cases fall in the 200 and 300 ranges.

Also keep an eye out for diabetes symptoms. When glucose can't get into your cells, it comes out in your urine, bringing water with it. As a result, you lose fluids and could experience:

- Unexplained weight loss
- Unusual thirst
- A frequent need to urinate
- Feelings of tiredness most of the time for no apparent reason

Other warning signs include:

- Cuts and bruises that heal slowly
- Tingling or numbness in your hands and feet
- Recurring skin, gum, or bladder infections

Traditional Treatment

If your diabetes test is positive, there are at least a dozen kinds of medication in four different classes that your doctor might prescribe:

- Drugs that make the pancreas secrete more insulin (sulfonylureas and meglitinides)
- Drugs that make your body more sensitive to insulin (thiazolidinediones)
- Drugs that decrease the amount of sugar your liver produces (biguanides)
- Drugs that delay the absorption of glucose (alpha-glucosidase inhibitors)

"Just 4 or 5 years ago, we had only drugs that boosted insulin secretion, but now we have these other categories," says James Rosenzweig, M.D., senior physician at the Joslin Diabetes Center in Boston. "Many of the pills work in combination, so if one works only partially, it's not a failure because we can add a second drug."

While doctors take side effects into account when they decide which class of drugs to prescribe, they also base their decision on your symptoms.

If you are overweight, you are probably insulin resistant, so your doctor will probably prescribe a medication that makes you more sensitive to the hormone, such as Avandia or Actos. If your sugars are very high (in the 200 or 300 range) and you're not overweight, you probably have a hard time secreting insulin, so your doctor might put you on a drug that stimulates your pancreas to secrete insulin, such as Glucotrol or Micronase.

Insulin shots are usually reserved for people with severe cases of type 2 diabetes. Insulin is injected, absorbed into the tissues underneath the skin, and circulated in the bloodstream. Injections in the stomach make insulin work faster, while injecting it into the upper arm or thigh slows down its effects.

Different kinds of insulin have different lengths and peaks of action in the body. Some cause blood sugar to drop quickly, while others have a solution added to them that slows their absorption.

People with diabetes usually start out able to treat their disease with lifestyle changes alone, but as they age and the disease progresses, they may have to start taking medication. Sooner or later, even the drugs may lose their effectiveness as the disease naturally progresses, Dr. Rosenzweig says. Eventually, you may need insulin or a combination of drugs and insulin.

Avoid Complications

Some shocking news: Only one-third of those with type 2 diabetes take their medication regularly.

"Diabetes involves a lot of regimentation, blood tests, and deciding what to eat and when to exercise," Dr. Rosenzweig says. "It takes a lot of work to do a good job with it. By ignoring all the regimentation, it's almost like people are denying they have the disease."

But not taking your medication means you're risking chronic high blood sugar, which could end up causing even more serious diseases in the future.

Tracking your blood sugar is the only way to know if you're treating your diabetes right. If your blood sugar stays consistently low, you can check it about three times a week. But if you have more trouble keeping it steady, your doctor will probably advise you to check it every day or even more than once a day.

Blood sugar levels can get too high if you don't follow a healthy diet or if you're sick or stressed. When your blood sugar is high, you may have headaches, blurred vision, feelings of thirst, the need to urinate often, or dry, itchy skin.

On the other hand, your blood sugar can get too low if you eat too little or nothing at all, take too much diabetes medicine, exercise too hard or long, or drink alcohol without eating. Then you might feel shaky, tired, hungry, confused, or nervous. When this happens, you

THE REZULIN FIASCO: HOW DID IT HAPPEN?

Rezulin entered the scene in March 1997 as one of the most promising oral drugs ever marketed to treat type 2 diabetes.

Put on a fast track for approval by the FDA because of its promise, it avoided much of the red tape often involved in gaining the agency's green light. It was designed to be used in addition to insulin or sulfonylureas to lower blood sugar by increasing the body's sensitivity to insulin.

By December 1997, with 600,000 people in the United States taking the drug, the FDA received reports that 2 percent of Rezulin users had mild elevations of liver enzymes, suggesting liver irritation.

So the FDA recommended that Rezulin users have liver function tests every 3 months and stop taking the drug if liver enzymes became too high or if they experienced symptoms of liver dysfunction, such as nausea, vomiting, abdominal pain, fatigue, loss of appetite, or dark urine.

Then, in early 1998, the agency learned that 150 more people had experienced liver trouble and that 3 in Japan had died. It then required liver testing *before* the drug was prescribed, every month for 6 months after starting the drug, and every other month for the rest of the first year on the drug. At the request of the FDA, the drug's manufacturer, Warner-Lambert, changed the drug's label four times over the next 3 years to include warnings for liver damage.

But reports of liver damage and deaths from the drug continued, and on March 21, 2000, the FDA asked Warner-Lambert to pull Rezulin from the market. By then, it had linked Rezulin to 89 reports of liver failure and 61 deaths. Consumer groups had lobbied for the drug's removal, claiming that Warner-Lambert knew Rezulin could cause liver damage before it even hit the market and that it withheld this information from the FDA. Some patients sued the drug maker.

The good news: The FDA says that two similar drugs, Avandia and Actos, are just as effective and are safer for the liver.

WOMAN TO WOMAN

Losing Weight Meant No More Symptoms

Jennifer Byers, 41, of Columbia, South Carolina, was diagnosed with diabetes in 1995. Despite her doctor's advice, she didn't change her lifestyle until 5 years later, when she couldn't ignore her symptoms any longer. Here's what she did.

When my diabetes symptoms got so bad I was experiencing heart palpitations, thirst that water just couldn't quench, and trips to the bathroom more than twice a night to urinate, I knew I had to make a change in my life.

So I went to the library to learn as much as I could about the disease. I pored through books, magazines, and medical journals and figured out what caused my diabetes: poor diet, obesity, and inactivity. I weighed 225 pounds at the time, was living on potato chips and pork chops, and wasn't getting any exercise. I knew my unhealthy lifestyle had to change.

First, I concentrated on getting more fiber and natural foods because I read that whole grains get absorbed slowly and help keep blood sugar levels steady. I also replaced red meat and ham for dinner with vegetable soup and ate lots of bean burritos with onions and fresh peppers, muffins sweetened with bananas, and fresh fruit. I even found the time, with two kids, to bake homemade whole wheat bread.

Finally, I was following all the nutrition advice I had known for years. Now, I was eating the squash, tomatoes, onions, and garlic from my garden instead of filling up on chips and baked goods from the grocery store.

I also knew I had to exercise, but I hated doing it. So I made my workouts as pleasant as possible. Instead of exercising outside in the middle of a hot South Carolina day, I get up at 5:00 A.M., when it's cool, dark, and quiet outside. I alternate walking and running for a mile and a half. I also take every opportunity to be more active all day. For instance, I run instead of walk up stairs and out to the mailbox.

In 3 weeks, my symptoms disappeared, and in 6 months, I lost 30 pounds and gained the energy diabetes had at first taken away.

need to eat or drink some simple carbohydrates, like ½ cup of a regular soft drink or fruit juice, 2 tablespoons of raisins, a few hard candies, or 1 tablespoon of sugar.

"Once you get the disease, the clock is ticking as to whether you get all the complications that typically occur 10 to 15 years after you're diagnosed," says Dr. Rosenzweig. "If you let your blood sugars chronically go into the 200 range without doing anything about it, it can cause serious problems later on, even though you might feel perfectly fine now." Those problems include heart disease, kidney disease, eye disease, peripheral vascular disease, nerve disease, amputations, and periodontal disease.

Beating—And Avoiding—Diabetes

A Finnish study found that all it may take for many people to significantly lower blood glucose levels is lifestyle changes, including exercise and a low-fat, high-fiber diet.

If your medical doctor doesn't suggest changing your diet and exercising to control your diabetes, seek advice from a dietitian, certified diabetes educator, or a naturopathic physician instead of going it alone, says Rita Bettenburg, N.D., associate professor at National College of Naturopathic Medicine in Portland, Oregon.

Even if you don't already have diabetes, these strategies could help you avoid the disease in the first place. If you have been diagnosed with it, they'll help you control your blood sugar and avoid complications.

Lose the Weight

Researchers have found that people who carry genes that make them prone to abdominal fat also carry genes that make them resistant to insulin. Also, doctors say high levels of abdominal fat, compared with total body fat, appear to induce insulin resistance.

According to one study, if your body mass index (BMI), which measures the amount of fat in your body, is higher than 27, you may be insulin resistant and at risk for diabetes. To calculate your BMI: Multiply your weight by 705. Divide that number by the square of your height in inches.

If you already have diabetes, losing just 10 percent of your overall weight may help keep the disease from progressing. But don't expect it to be easy. For reasons not completely understood, doctors have noticed that people with diabetes have a harder time losing weight than those without, says Diane Krieger, M.D., endocrinologist and director of the Diabetes Care Program in South Miami. Some diabetes medications also make weight loss difficult. Ways to help drop pounds include:

Practice the pyramid. Refresh your memory of what a healthy diet looks like by following the USDA Food Guide Pyramid. Eat balanced meals of grains, vegetables, fruit, protein and dairy, with only small amounts of fat, fried food, and sweets.

Get three squares. People with diabetes have to pay special attention to eating about the same amount of food at about the same time every day to keep their blood sugar levels from fluctuating wildly, says Ann Zerr, M.D., clinical director of the National Center of Excellence in Women's Health at Indiana University School of Medicine in Indianapolis. If you're on insulin, your blood sugar could drop to dangerous levels if you skip meals. Skipping also won't save you calories because you're very likely to overeat at your next meal.

If you don't have diabetes, eating regularly without skipping meals keeps your metabolism going strong and your weight down, so you may lower your risk of getting diabetes.

Watch your carbs. Because carbohydrates raise blood sugar levels faster than fat and protein, it's important to eat about the same amount of carbohydrates at every meal—about 50 percent of your total calories. Carbohydrates include sugar, starch, fruits, and some vegetables. For an easy way to sum up your meal, check that carbohydrates take up half or less of your plate. The rest of your meal should be composed of proteins and fat.

Reach for complex carbohydrates, such as whole grains. They're usually low in calories and full of vitamins, minerals, and fiber. They should make up the bulk of your carbohydrates. Whole grains and other high-fiber foods are better choices than refined carbohydrates. That means opting for bran cereal, cooked beans and peas, whole grain bread, fruits, and vegetables instead of white flour, white bread, and white rice. One study of almost 36,000 women found those who ate more than 23 grams of fiber a day reduced their risk of diabetes 22 percent, compared with women who ate 15 grams or less a day. Want to eat enough fiber today? Try 1/2 cup of All-Bran cereal for breakfast and 1 cup of black bean soup for lunch. Bingo! You've just gotten 27 grams.

Have just a trace. Studies show that certain foods containing the trace mineral vanadium help your body use glucose, thus maintaining steady blood sugar levels and managing diabetes.

So reach for these foods: skim milk, gelatin, Grape-Nuts, lentils, navy beans, lobster, vegetable oils, radishes, potatoes, turnip greens, squash, lettuce, and hazelnuts.

Don't be too sweet. For many years, people with diabetes were told to avoid sugar because it would raise their blood glucose levels more than other carbohydrates. But research has shown that this is not true. Although eating a piece of cake will raise your glucose level, so will eating corn on the cob or lima beans.

There's no reason for people with diabetes to avoid sugar completely, but moderation is the rule. Eat too much and you may send your blood glucose level up higher than expected. You'll also gain weight and fill up on empty calories without getting the vitamins and minerals your body needs. When you do eat sweets, eat fewer carbohydrates the rest of the day. If you'd like a little sweetness without the calories, try artificial sweeteners, such as aspartame or saccharin. For baking, try the newest artificial sweetener, acesulfame potassium (Sweet One).

Watch your fat and salt. People with diabetes have to be especially careful not to get too much fat in their diet since they're already at high risk for heart disease. If they also have high blood pressure, they should avoid eating too much table salt and salty foods. That means going lightly on things like pickles, bacon, cheese, salad dressing, and canned soups because high blood pressure increases their risk of heart and kidney disease. They should try to keep their daily sodium intake at 2,400 milligrams or less. If they also have kidney disease, their daily

BLAME IT ON HORMONES
Polycystic Ovary Syndrome

An alarming number of women—an estimated 6 to 10 percent—have polycystic ovary syndrome (PCOS), and many don't even know it. It's the most common endocrine syndrome in premenopausal women and the leading cause of infertility in the United States.

"The current thinking is that PCOS is a kind of unique insulin resistance syndrome," says Rose Christian, M.D., an endocrine research fellow at the National Institutes of Health in Bethesda, Maryland.

When a woman has PCOS, insulin stimulates extra testosterone production in her ovaries and liver. Many women with PCOS are insulin resistant or glucose intolerant (so they have excess insulin in their blood), and they have a higher risk of developing diabetes than the general population. In fact, one in 10 women with PCOS develops diabetes by age 40.

Some of this extra insulin finds its way to the ovaries, where it attaches to receptors and directs the ovaries to increase their production of testosterone.

In the liver, the extra insulin lowers sex hormone binding globulin (SHBG). Normally, testosterone binds to SHBG and is rendered, well, impotent. But the lower the amount of SHBG, the more active testosterone is available, resulting in:

➤ Irregular menstrual periods

➤ Inability to ovulate

sodium intake should be 2,000 milligrams or less.

Stop after one glass of wine. Because alcohol is a toxin, your liver wants to clear it from the blood quickly. But this can be a problem if you have diabetes. Normally, when your blood glucose level starts to drop, your liver steps in and sends glucose out into the blood. But your liver won't send out any glucose until it clears all the alcohol in your blood. Thus, drinking may

> ❥ Hair growth on the face
>
> ❥ Acne

More than 60 percent of women with PCOS are also obese, with a body mass index of 30 or more. Some doctors say excessive testosterone causes the obesity, but others disagree, pointing out that European women with PCOS are less likely to be overweight.

Women often develop PCOS at puberty, but many don't know they have it until their twenties or even thirties. In the past, when young women went to their doctors complaining of irregular periods, they were usually put on a birth control pill to trigger monthly menstruation. So they often wouldn't find out they had PCOS until they went off the Pill and stopped having any periods or couldn't get pregnant because they weren't ovulating.

"There's been an assumption for a long time that it's normal to have irregular periods in adolescence," says Dr. Christian. "But now, we're starting to understand that it's not normal and that this may be an early manifestation of PCOS and other endocrine abnormalities."

Testing involves a physical exam and blood tests to exclude other health problems. Hormones and medication can treat facial hair and acne. If you're not trying to get pregnant, your doctor will probably prescribe birth control pills to regulate your periods. If you are trying to get pregnant, you'll need hormones to help you ovulate and conceive. Treatment also includes regular exercise and maintaining a healthy weight.

snack before you go to sleep. Good choices include graham crackers, a piece of toast, a small bowl of cereal, a piece of fruit, and a piece of bread and cheese.

Keep Your Heart Pumping

When you begin a spinning class or other aerobic activity, your body produces more glucose to give your muscles energy to continue moving. As a result, your pancreas secretes more insulin. Exercise also makes you more sensitive to the insulin already in your cells, so you're better able to convert glucose into energy.

If you're on insulin or diabetes medication and you're starting an exercise program, let your doctor know. After exercising, you may be able to get by with a lower dose of medication or even go off insulin entirely. Here's how to get the most out of exercise.

Work it into your daily routine. A half-hour of activity most days can help prevent diabetes, Dr. Zerr says, and that doesn't mean 30 minutes of grueling aerobics. A walk also works, whether it's for 30 minutes straight or broken up into three 10-minute sessions throughout the day.

But to keep blood sugar levels steady, especially if you're taking insulin, try to exercise at about the same time every day, Dr. Rosenzweig suggests.

If you don't have time for 30 minutes a day, find little ways to be more active. Get up to change the channel, park and walk into the bank or restaurant instead of using the drive-thru

lead to low blood sugar, especially on an empty stomach, after exercising, or while you're taking insulin or diabetes medication. Also, alcohol is full of nutritionally empty calories, which could make it harder to lose weight if that's part of your diabetes-control plan. If you do drink, stick with only one—and try light beer, dry wine, or a mixture of alcohol and diet soda.

Eat a bedtime snack. If your blood sugar tends to get too low overnight, have a nutritious

HORMONES THROUGH HISTORY

The Discovery of Insulin

People have suffered from diabetes for 3,500 years, but no one pointed to insulin as the culprit until 1910, when an Edinburgh scientist named Sharpey-Shafer theorized that those with diabetes were missing one chemical in their pancreas. He named that chemical "insulin." Another scientist named R. C. Paulesco found that an extract from the pancreas lowered the blood sugar of dogs.

During the summer of 1922, a team of researchers at the University of Toronto proved that removing the pancreas gave dogs diabetes. They successfully extracted fluid from the islet cells of healthy dogs and injected it into dogs with diabetes. They found the dogs' symptoms disappeared. Later that year, they extracted pure insulin from the pancreas of cattle and gave it to a teenager with diabetes, whose symptoms improved dramatically.

The four scientists involved in the discovery were Frederick Banting, Charles Best, J. B. Collip, and J. J. R. Macleod. Banting and Macleod received the Nobel Prize in medicine in 1923, and they shared the prize money with the two other scientists. By then, insulin was widely available and had saved many lives.

Before this discovery, the only treatment for diabetes was a strict low-carbohydrate, low-sugar diet. Even so, people with diabetes lived only about a year after diagnosis.

Until 1978, most insulin came from animals, mainly cattle and pigs. It wasn't until 1978 that researchers manufactured human insulin, the first human protein to be made through biotechnology.

Don't let your sugar get too low. Plan snacks according to your exercise routine. If you walk, bike, or golf more than an hour after meals, eat a carbohydrate snack before your workout. Six ounces of fruit juice or half a plain bagel will do. If your workout is more aerobically intense, have a little more, such as half a meat sandwich or a cup of low-fat milk.

Calm Down

When we're stressed, we go into the fight-or-flight mode. Our bodies release stress hormones like adrenaline, and our livers send in extra glucose to give our muscles energy, raising blood sugar levels. In people with diabetes, insulin may not always be able to get the extra energy into the cells; thus, blood sugar levels can rise. But this effect varies greatly among individuals, with some experiencing *lower* blood sugar levels.

"If you have diabetes, the major effect of emotional stress is on behavior," says Dr. Rosenzweig. "Stress can affect your ability to eat right, exercise, and take your medication correctly, which results in uncontrolled glucose levels," he explains.

Just the diagnosis could stress you out because it involves changing your lifestyle and raises concerns about complications.

You'll know that you're stressed if you notice changes in your sleep patterns, appetite, energy, sex drive, or work habits. You might withdraw from friends and family, experience

window, and take the stairs instead of the elevator.

Build muscle. Lifting weights may also help control or prevent diabetes. Exercising your muscles increases the amount of glucose converted to energy. Lift weights two or three times a week, with at least a day of rest between sessions.

panic attacks, lose interest in things you usually enjoy, lash out at people, drink alcohol, or take drugs.

Talk to a doctor if you feel overwhelmed by stress. For more information on coping with stress, see Fight or Flight: The Stress Hormones on page 52.

Go for Alternatives

While diet and exercise are the two most important ways to control and prevent diabetes, you may also find help in supplements and herbs. But don't try them alone; get help from a naturopathic doctor, says Dr. Bettenburg. You'll need someone to monitor your response to these treatments. And make sure you check with your medical doctor about any supplements or herbs you take because they can interfere with your medications. Some that are suggested for those with diabetes or who are at high risk of the disease include:

Gymnema sylvestre. This Indian herb boosts insulin production, according to animal studies, and a drop of tincture on your tongue can stop sugar cravings, says David Winston, an herbalist in Washington, New Jersey, and founding member of the American Herbalists Guild.

Chromium. An essential nutrient, chromium assists in glucose metabolism. One study found that 200 micrograms of supplemental chromium a day can help to control glucose and increase the amount of insulin that binds to your cells. Women with severe cases of diabetes might need a higher dose, says Michael Janson, M.D., of Arlington, Massachusetts, author of *Dr. Janson's New Vitamin Revolution*.

Cinnamon. Researchers at the USDA Agricultural Research Service laboratory set out to find natural ways to lower blood sugar by testing some of the plants and spices used in folk medicine. Of 50 plant extracts that were tested, cinnamon—the same spice you find in your cupboard—made it easiest for cells to use insulin. Clinical trials that may lead to a patent of the cinnamon extract began in 2001. In the meantime, Winston suggests stirring $\frac{1}{4}$ to 1 teaspoon of ground cinnamon into your orange juice, coffee, or oatmeal every day.

Bitter melon. A vegetable that looks like a shriveled cucumber, bitter melon is used as traditional medicine in China, India, and Africa to lower blood sugar. It's available in Asian grocery stores, and you can use it in soup, tea, or a stir-fry with vegetables and chicken or tofu. Keep in mind that it tastes like its name, says Winston. Don't use it, however, if you have low blood sugar or if you are pregnant.

Vitamins C and E. Both antioxidants halt a process called glycosylation, where sugar reacts with protein, altering its structure so it can be used by the body. This is what's thought to cause complications such as blindness, kidney disease, and nerve damage, says Janson.

Vitamin C also prevents glucose already inside your cells from being converted to sorbitol, a sugar alcohol that can't be used for energy. As a result, vitamin C lowers blood sugar levels, blood cholesterol levels, and thus your risk for complications.

Doctors also think vitamin E helps keep insulin receptor sites working properly, says Janson.

Try taking 1,000 to 4,000 milligrams a day of vitamin C and 400 to 800 international units of vitamin E, he says. But tell your doctor first, especially if you are already taking aspirin or an anticoagulant (blood-thinning) medication, such as warfarin (Coumadin). Vitamin E also acts like a blood thinner.

Taking more than 2,000 milligrams of vitamin C might cause diarrhea. Those with late-stage diabetes shouldn't take either because they could cause kidney failure.

ADDISON'S DISEASE

Addison's disease, also called adrenal cortical insufficiency, is an uncommon disease involving the adrenal glands. The adrenal glands produce many hormones, some of which are involved in metabolizing carbohydrates and fats. One in 100,000 people gets the disease each year.

Addison's disease may be caused by tuberculosis and autoimmune disease. These days, doctors can treat tuberculosis better than they used to, so there are fewer cases of TB-related Addison's. More commonly, people get the disease when their immune systems treat the body as a foreign invader and attack it, explains Lila A. Wallis, M.D., M.A.C.P., clinical professor of medicine at Weill Medical College of Cornell University in New York City.

In this case, the immune system attacks the adrenal cortex, the outside portion of the adrenal glands.

When destroyed, the adrenal cortex can't secrete the hormones aldosterone and cortisol. Aldosterone regulates salt and water levels, and cortisol helps regulate blood sugar levels under stress, as well as the amount of water in the body.

Without enough aldosterone and cortisol, people who have Addison's feel weak or tired, dizzy, irritable, or depressed. They lose their appetite, lose weight, have low blood pressure, and crave salty food. They may also notice their skin becoming darker, especially on scars, elbows, knees, knuckles, toes, and lips. Women may have irregular menstrual periods. The autoimmune mechanism is also responsible for type 1 diabetes, and some people may develop both.

Symptoms of Addison's disease progress slowly, and some women might not know they have it until an illness makes it worse, a condition called an Addisonian crisis. Symptoms include severe vomiting, diarrhea, and sudden pain in the lower back, abdomen, or legs. Dehydration, low blood pressure, and loss of consciousness follow. Without immediate treatment, it could be fatal.

Treatment involves replacing the lacking hormones with medication.

Alpha lipoic acid. This antioxidant helps your body reprocess antioxidants like vitamins C and E so they stick around longer to do their good deeds. It also reduces the risk of diabetes complications, such as nerve pain and eye disease. Dr. Janson recommends 300 to 1,000 milligrams a day. Don't take more than 800 milligrams a day for more than 4 months.

Give Yourself Time

Whether you're trying to eat healthier, exercise more, or stop stressing out, you won't be able to get rid of your old habits tomorrow. Give yourself at least 6 months to gradually become healthier, Dr. Bettenburg says. Even if you're not eating and exercising as well as you can by then, acknowledge the progress you've made and keep at it.

The good news: A study found that baby boomers are more proactive in treating their diabetes through diet and exercise than their parents were. They're also good about asking their doctors for alternative ways to treat their disease.

The Thyroid:
Energy for Everything

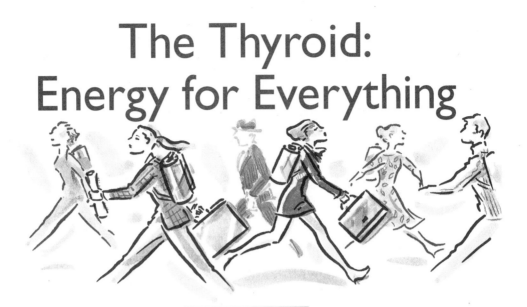

Let's list the modern woman's litany of complaints: I'm too tired. I'm too fat. My cholesterol is too high.

You could blame bad living, but you might also blame your supergland, the thyroid.

"Your thyroid gland produces hormones that affect every organ, every tissue, and every cell in the body," says David Brownstein, M.D., associate clinical professor of medicine at Wayne State University in Bloomfield, Michigan, and author of *The Miracle of Natural Hormones*.

Yet by the time we're 50, one in ten of us will have signs of a failing thyroid. We just won't know it.

This doesn't have to be you. By paying attention to your body and being assertive with your doctor, you can make sure you're not kept in the dark. And even if there's nothing wrong with your thyroid now, there are things you can do to keep it healthy as you age.

Inside the Thyroid Gland

The thyroid is a butterfly-shaped gland located in front of the windpipe at the base of the neck. It releases hormones called thyroxine (T4) and triiodothyronine (T3) into your blood. These hormones help regulate your heart rate, body temperature, and metabolism, including how efficiently you burn calories.

But like every gland, the thyroid doesn't work alone. The pituitary gland, located deep within your brain, acts like a thermostat, constantly tracking the amount of thyroid hormone in your blood. If there's too little, the pituitary releases thyroid stimulating hormone (TSH), which signals the thyroid to make more thyroid hormone. Once the pituitary senses that your hormone levels are restored, it slows its production of TSH. If your thyroid gland produces too much thyroid hormone, the pituitary sends less TSH to the gland in an attempt to turn down the heat, so to speak.

Chronic levels of too much or too little thyroid hormone interfere with the proper function of every major organ. Generally, the thyroid gland causes problems in two different ways.

Hypothyroidism, or not enough thyroid hormone. This slows your body down and can trigger a slew of symptoms as long as a 5-year-

BLAME IT ON HORMONES
Winter Birthdays and Weight Gain

We all know that lifestyle and genetics play an important role in whether we pile on the pounds as we age. Now it looks like we may also be able to blame the weather.

Researchers have long known that bigger babies are more likely than smaller ones to become obese in adulthood. But a recent study suggests the connection exists in men, at least, if they were big babies (more than 9 pounds, 8 ounces) *and* were born following a particularly cold winter, says researcher James B. Young, M.D., of Northwestern University in Chicago. The effect was less pronounced in women, he said.

He and fellow researcher David Phillips of the University of Southampton in Great Britain examined the birth records of 1,165 men and 585 women born between 1920 and 1930 in Hertfordshire, England. Overall, 20 percent of the women and 11 percent of the men were obese. But when the researchers divided the participants into two groups—those born following mild winters and those born following cold winters—they found that people born following cold weather were more likely to be obese.

Though researchers aren't sure why weight is linked to weather, they speculate that the cold may set limits on how well the thyroid gland works. The involuntary nervous system of people born after it's cold may be programmed differently. That would influence thyroid function as well as how certain organs in the body metabolize thyroid hormone, explains Dr. Young.

old's birthday wish list, including unexplained fatigue, hair loss, weight gain, depression, cold hands and feet, dry skin, low body temperature, low blood pressure, menstrual irregularities, infertility, PMS, osteoporosis, sugar cravings, hypoglycemia, constipation, forgetfulness, muscle cramps and spasms, problems digesting fats and oils, respiratory infections, lowered resistance to colds and flu, migraines, and chronic headaches.

More than half of the 11 million Americans who have underactive thyroids don't know it. What's most scary is that, left untreated, hypothyroidism can raise cholesterol levels and increase the risk of heart disease.

The most common cause of hypothyroidism is an immune system dysfunction called *Hashimoto's thyroiditis*, where your body produces antibodies that attack the thyroid gland as if it were a foreign substance, damaging it so it no longer produces enough hormones.

Conventional treatment calls for replacing the missing hormone with a daily tablet of levothyroxine, a synthetic form of T4, which you usually need to take for the rest of your life.

Hyperthyroidism, or too much thyroid hormone. Less common, hyperthyroidism affects about one million Americans—most of them women in their thirties and forties. Too much thyroid hormone sends the body into overdrive, causing symptoms such as nervousness, hand tremors, palpitations, weight loss, insomnia, shortness of breath (especially with exercise), increased sweating, increased appetite, fatigue, muscle weakness, eye irritation, and bulging eyes.

Hyperthyroidism is most often caused by Graves' disease, which tends to run in families. Like Hashimoto's thyroiditis, Graves' is an autoimmune condition. But instead of antibodies destroying thyroid tissue, they trigger *increased* hormone production. Sometimes a lump or nodule within the thyroid gland can also cause your thyroid to pump out too much hormone.

Because hyperthyroidism can be life-threatening, even holistic doctors generally recommend conventional treatments for it. "The best conventional treatment for hyperthyroidism is oral doses of radioactive iodine," says Andrew Weil, M.D., director of the integrative medicine program and clinical professor of internal medicine at the University of Arizona College of Medicine in Tucson. "While this sounds frightful, it's relatively safe (most of the radioactivity is excreted in the urine within 48 hours) and quite effective."

Once taken, radioactive iodine goes from the stomach into the bloodstream and ultimately to the overactive thyroid gland, where it stays long enough to damage some of the thyroid cells and slow things down. Most people get well in 3 to 6 months after just one dose. Those who remain hyperthyroid are usually given a second and sometimes a third dose. One of the consequences of treatment: Most people who receive radioactive iodine end up with an underactive thyroid, which means you have to take thyroid hormones for the rest of your life.

Other conventional treatments include antithyroid drugs, which can cause skin rashes and liver problems, and removing part of the thyroid gland.

Preventing Thyroid Disease

The likelihood of developing a thyroid disorder increases with age, with 17 percent of women experiencing a failing thyroid by age 60. Other factors that increase your risk include a family history of thyroid or autoimmune disease, pregnancy, x-ray therapy to the head and neck for cancer, and high cholesterol.

Though experts aren't sure exactly why our thyroids tend to fail as we get older, there are measures you can take to reduce your risk.

Reduce stress. Without a doubt, stress reduction improves the entire hormonal system, says Joseph Mercola, D.O., who runs the Optimal Wellness Center in Schaumburg, Illinois. Chronic stress can impair the adrenal glands, which inhibits thyroid function. The fact that both former president Bush and his wife were diagnosed with Graves' disease may be an indication of the stress of public life.

"The single most effective relaxation technique I know is conscious regulation of breath," says Dr. Weil.

Place the tip of your tongue against the ridge of tissue just behind your upper front teeth and *keep it there through the entire exercise.* You will be exhaling through your mouth around your tongue. Try pursing your lips slightly if this seems awkward.

- First, exhale completely through your mouth, making a "whoosh" sound.
- Next, close your mouth and inhale quietly through your nose to a mental count of four.
- Hold your breath for a count of seven.
- Exhale completely through your mouth, making a whoosh sound to a count of eight. This is one breath.

Now, inhale again and repeat the cycle three more times for a total of four breaths.

Eat right. Wellness starts with a healthy diet. That means plenty of organic fruits and veggies because they're free of pesticides that can interfere with thyroid function, says Carol Roberts, M.D., a holistic physician and director of Wellness Works in Tampa. Whole grains and lean protein also supply the amino acid tyrosine, needed for thyroid hormone production, she adds. Limit sugar and refined carbohydrates, like cakes, cookies, and white breads, which can overstimulate the adrenal glands.

"All my patients take basic multivitamins, including vitamins C and E, all the B vitamins, and beta-carotene," says Dr. Roberts. Because our food is often deficient in minerals, make sure your vitamin supplement includes minerals, too. "Balanced minerals are crucial to the proper function of the whole body," she says.

Go slow on soy. There's evidence that consuming more than 8 grams of soy daily from products like soy protein powder, soy milk, tofu, and supplements—all of which are high in isoflavones—may cause hypothyroidism. "I would also advise people to avoid nonfermented and nonsprouted soy products, since we really don't know how much is safe to eat," says Dr. Mercola, who has a Web site at www.mercola.com that contains more information on thyroid disease.

Soy is not the ideal supplement or superfood that we have been led to believe, says Dr. Mercola. Many people are allergic to soy, and a high intake of soy can also impair digestion, he adds.

Drink bottled water. Fluoride in tap water and trace amounts of toxic chemicals may trigger thyroid problems or worsen the risk, says Dr. Roberts. "Most cities fluoridate their drinking water, and it is almost impossible to find toothpaste that doesn't contain fluoride, so we're getting a lot. This may be a hidden cause of hypothyroidism." Like a mineral version of musical chairs, fluoride may compete with iodine for places to bind within the body. By decreasing the body's access to iodine, fluoride may ultimately lower thyroid function, Dr. Roberts adds. In fact, scientists in the late 1920s were the first to figure out that fluoride slowed thyroid function and use it to treat hyperthyroidism.

WOMAN TO WOMAN
Her Doctor Said It Was Stress

Flagging energy and a host of chronic symptoms made Cathy Uselton, 39, an editor and Web master from Choctaw, Oklahoma, suspect something was wrong. Despite numerous visits to the doctor, it took 3 years to get her diagnosis of hypothyroidism. Her advice: If you suspect something is wrong, be persistent.

I began having symptoms when I was 34, after the birth of my second child. I went to my doctor off and on for almost 3 years with different symptoms—recurring infections, sore throats that would last for 3 to 4 weeks at a time, pain in my joints, fatigue, and headaches.

He wasn't an arrogant or bad sort. He was just very close to retirement age, and I don't think he was on top of his game anymore.

He would pat me on the back and say, "Well, you're obviously a fine, healthy woman." In the meantime, my hair became like straw and began to fall out. I also began to have severe trouble concentrating and thinking. I'd forget my home phone number. At least 10 times a day, I'd go into a room and forget why I was there. One day in the car on the way to the bank, I didn't remember where I was going or how to get home—and I've lived in my hometown all my life. The doctor said I had stress and needed to take a few days off.

It also seemed like I was losing my hearing. When I was with a group of people, I couldn't hear what they were

Stop smoking. We all know that smoking can damage the lungs. Now comes new evidence that it may cause thyroid disease as well, notes Dr. Mercola. A study of 132 pairs of twins showed that smoking can have negative effects on the endocrine system, causing a three- to fivefold increase in the risk of all types of thyroid disease. The association was most pronounced in people with autoimmune disorders (Graves' disease and Hashimoto's thyroiditis), although

saying. Everything sounded like mumbling. On top of that, my ears were ringing 8 to 12 times a day. It was time for another visit to the doctor.

When I got there, the nurse took my blood pressure. I've always had low blood pressure—around 100/60—and 80/50 wasn't unusual for me. But this time, my pressure was 160/100.

The doctor read my chart, listened to my symptoms, and promptly wrote me prescriptions for an antihistamine and decongestant (he said my ear troubles were caused by allergies, even though I didn't have any fluid in my ears). Then he left the room. He never said a thing about my blood pressure. At that point, I decided I needed a new doctor.

My new doctor's response upon hearing my symptoms was an immediate "We've got to get you a blood test to check for thyroid and liver enzymes!"

My TSH test came back 40. Based on that number, my doctor said my thyroid probably hadn't worked in 2 to 3 years.

I've been on thyroid medication for 2 years now. I still have some problems, especially with my weight, sleep, and mood, but I'm feeling much better than I was before I was diagnosed. I have much more energy. I work full time, and I still have energy to spend with my husband and children when I get home most nights. Our weekends are a lot more fun now! As my husband says, "It's wonderful to have my wife back."

there was still a strong association for those with nonautoimmune thyroid disorders.

Change your bedtime. Sleep restores the immune system and quiets our often overstimulated adrenal glands. But it helps to time it right. "Remember that for most of human existence, our bodies have been tied to the biorhythms of the sun," says Dr. Mercola. "During certain times of the night, our bodies are programmed to eliminate toxins and produce melatonin, a

hormone that helps us sleep. Both help support healthy thyroid function."

Avoid mercury dental fillings. Mercury is a common cause of hypothyroidism, says Dr. Mercola. "Amalgam fillings are 50 percent mercury, and they are only inches away from the thyroid." Ask your dentist to use nonmetal fillings. However, be careful to select a dentist who is properly trained to do this procedure, or you may run into complications, says Dr. Mercola. And if you're at risk for hypothyroidism, consider having the existing amalgam fillings removed from your teeth by a properly trained and experienced "holistic" dentist.

Getting Diagnosed

Symptoms of thyroid disorders are often subtle and easily dismissed. Along with our doctors, we tend to chalk them up to stress, aging, or menopause. In fact, more than half of American women over 40 have experienced at least three symptoms of a thyroid disorder, yet 75 percent of them haven't bothered to discuss them with their doctors.

"Even when women arm themselves with a list of symptoms, they're frequently told that they're stressed, depressed, PMSing, or just getting older," says Mary Shomon, author of *Living Well with Hypothyroidism*, who founded a patient-advocacy newsletter and Web site after she was diagnosed with hypothyroidism in 1996.

All this means that a thyroid problem can fester for years before it's finally diagnosed. An Internet poll asked more than 2,000 thyroid pa-

Key Thyroid Function Tests

Test Name	Normal Range	What It Means
TSH (thyroid stimulating hormone)	0.4–2.0	Less than 0.4 can indicate hyperthyroidism. More than 2.0 suggests hypothyroidism.
Total T4	4.5–12.5	Less than 4.5 can indicate an underactive thyroid when TSH is also elevated. More than 12.5 can indicate hyperthyroidism. Low T4 with low TSH may suggest a pituitary problem.
Free T4	0.7–2.0	Less than 0.7 indicates hypothyroidism.
T3	80–220	Less than 80 can indicate hypothyroidism.

tients how long it took them to get a diagnosis and found that it took more than 2 years for 52 percent of them.

So expect an accurate diagnosis to take some patience and perseverance on your part. The rewards are worth it. "It's impossible to achieve optimal health with a poorly functioning thyroid," says Dr. Brownstein. To help you get the right diagnosis, experts suggest these approaches.

Write it all down. List your symptoms in a journal, calendar, or notebook to make it easier for you to communicate your risk factors to your doctor. It also serves as an aid in getting a proper diagnosis, says Shomon. Her Web site, http://thyroid.about.com, features an easy-to-use symptom checklist.

Take your temperature. Although conventional doctors rely almost exclusively on blood tests to diagnose thyroid problems, basal temperature measurements are a far more accurate indication of hypothyroidism, says Dr. Mercola. However, temperature readings are not as accurate as free hormone levels, he adds.

Calculate your basal temperature by averaging your first morning temperature for three days. If you're still menstruating, take your temperature on days 2, 3, and 4 of your cycle. (Day 1 is the first day of your period.) To do this, place an easy-to-read, old-fashioned glass thermometer on your bedside table (make sure to shake it down before you go to bed). When you wake up, place the thermometer in your armpit and leave it there for 10 minutes without getting out of bed. If your average temperature is 97.8°F or less, you may have hypothyroidism.

Get tested. New guidelines issued by the American Thyroid Association say everyone should be screened for thyroid problems every 5 years, starting at age 35, with a simple blood test that measures the amount of TSH. (To understand what those test numbers mean, see "Key Thyroid Function Tests.")

Question the test. While testing is a good place to start, many holistic physicians say there is often no relationship between TSH test results and how people actually feel. "For every patient with an elevated TSH level who is hypothyroid, I must treat four others whose TSH is normal but whose temperature and clinical symptoms are consistent with decreased thyroid function," says Dr. Mercola.

Other doctors echo this experience.

After analyzing symptoms in hundreds of patients, Dr. Roberts found a strong correlation between a TSH value of 2.0 or more and a diagnosis for hypothyroidism. Most conventional doctors look for the TSH value to be over 5.5 when diagnosing hypothyroidism, he adds. So ask your doctor for the specific TSH value of your test.

You can also ask to have your free thyroid hormones levels tested. Tests for free T4 and T3 measure the hormones your cells are actually using. In traditional medicine, doctors use *total* T4 and T3 tests, which show only the level of hormones bound together with protein in the blood, says Dr. Mercola.

Find the right doc. "Many traditional physicians would rather believe a lab test than the patient sitting in front of them," says Dr. Mercola. Know when it's time to move on and find a doctor who's sympathetic to your concerns. Interview candidates over the phone first. Ask if they're willing to prescribe natural hormones or recommend alternative as well as conventional treatments for thyroid problems. Also ask if they're willing to base a diagnosis on more than just your TSH levels. For leads, check out the Thyroid Top Docs Directory at www.thyroid-info.com, a state-by-state listing of doctors recommended by their patients.

Natural Hormone Solutions

Once you've been diagnosed with a thyroid disorder, it's likely that

WILSON'S SYNDROME

In the early 1990s, E. Denis Wilson, M.D., developed a theory that major stress, such as divorce, illness, surgery, or childbirth, could cause changes in the thyroid hormones and slow the body down. As a result, body temperature drops, which is normal.

But for some people, he hypothesized, their temperature remains low even after the stress passes. This causes nearly all the enzymes in the body to function less effectively and can trigger nearly 60 kinds of hypothyroid-like symptoms, ranging from food cravings and irritability to acid indigestion and weight gain. The treatment for this condition, which he dubbed Wilson's syndrome, is a special form of T3 thyroid hormone replacement.

Before you chalk up your symptoms to Wilson's syndrome, however, consider statements from the American Thyroid Association, which says that there is no scientific evidence to support Wilson's theories. Its reasoning:

- The proposed basis for the syndrome is inconsistent with well-known and widely accepted facts about thyroid hormone production, metabolism, and action.

- The diagnosis of Wilson's syndrome is based on an incorrect definition of normal body temperature: 98.6°F. A study published in the *Journal of the American Medical Association* found that the average temperature of healthy persons at 8:00 A.M. is 97.6°. More than 50 percent of the temperatures measured in the study were less than 98.6°.

- The typical adult experiences at least one of the complaints attributed to Wilson's syndrome every 4 to 6 days.

- In the early 1990s, the state of Florida received complaints from several doctors about Dr. Wilson's questionable treatment of patients. Faced with a lawsuit, Dr. Wilson agreed not to practice medicine for 6 months. As of 2000, he had not yet returned to active medical practice but instead runs the for-profit Wilson's Syndrome Foundation.

your doctor will prescribe medication—typically, a synthetic form of thyroxine. Your thyroid levels come back to normal and your symptoms evaporate. End of story, right?

If only.

A more common scenario is that you've been taking one of the popular levothyroxine sodium thyroid replacement drugs—Levoxyl, Synthroid, Eltroxin—and your TSH is in the normal range . . . according to your doctor.

"But you still have symptoms. You're still not feeling well. You're having a tough time losing weight. You may be struggling with low-grade depression, hair loss, fatigue, or that hard-to-concentrate feeling many thyroid patients refer to as brain fog," says Shomon, who receives hundreds of e-mails each week from women who share the same frustrating situation.

There are a number of natural approaches that can complement (or sometimes replace) conventional treatments and help you feel better.

Consider natural thyroid replacement. If you're taking a synthetic hormone, such as Synthroid, but are still bothered by symptoms like forgetfulness, depression, or fatigue, ask your doctor about natural thyroid hormone replacement, says Dr. Mercola. Armour, the desiccated natural hormone product derived from pig glands, is a mixture of T3 and T4 and supplies the entire range of thyroid hormones.

A study published in the *New England Journal of Medicine* showed that patients with hypothyroidism who were treated with both T4 and T3 thyroid hormones improved in mood and performed better on cognitive tests than patients treated with T4 alone.

Often prescribed by natural practitioners, Armour has been around for 100 years and is regulated by the FDA, which considers it safe and effective.

Unfortunately, most doctors are taught in medical school that synthetic hormones are

better because it's easier to measure their levels in the blood, says Dr. Roberts.

But you can allay that fear by taking Armour twice a day, says Dr. Mercola, which helps stabilize the blood level of the more biologically active T3.

The most common starting dose for patients with hypothyroidism is 45 milligrams of Armour thyroid, taken after breakfast and dinner.

Supplement with kelp. Norwegian kelp is rich in iodine and trace minerals the body needs to produce thyroxine, but its use is controversial. "It seems that for every alternative practitioner you find who recommends you take iodine or kelp for your thyroid, there's one who disagrees," says Shomon, who interviewed hundreds of experts for her book.

Why the controversy? For people with autoimmune thyroid disorders, supplementing with iodine is akin to throwing gasoline on a fire.

And some experts maintain that we get enough iodine in our diets. At the same time, however, results from the National Health and Nutrition Examination Survey show the percentage of Americans with low iodine intake has quadrupled in the last 20 years. Currently, about 12 percent of the U.S. population is iodine deficient.

To see if you're deficient in iodine, paint a patch of tincture of iodine the size of a half-dollar on your belly. The brown discoloration should last for about 24 hours. If it disappears faster, you may be iodine deficient, says Dr. Mercola, who was recently diagnosed with hypothyroidism he believes is related to an iodine deficiency. Tincture of iodine is available at many pharmacies and health food stores.

Dr. Mercola recommends 5 grams of kelp a day if you're taking tablets or capsules. Or you can sprinkle loose, dried seaweed on food as a seasoning or salt substitute. Use about 1 ounce a week. If you have high blood pressure or heart

A THYROID BOOST FROM YOGA

The shoulder stand is a yoga pose that can help your thyroid function more efficiently. Work up to holding this position for 30 seconds to 1 minute daily.

- Lie flat on your back with your arms along your sides and your palms down.
- Raise your legs at the hips to a vertical position.
- Next, raise your hips so your chin rests on your chest. Support yourself by keeping your elbows and upper arms on the floor. Your hands should be at your hips with thumbs in front and fingers in back.
- Stretch your torso and legs as straight and tall as possible. At the same time, keep your neck and shoulders flat on the floor.
- Breathe normally and hold the pose for 30 seconds to 1 minute, or for as long as is comfortable.
- End the pose by first slowly lowering your knees toward your head, then lowering your legs to the floor.

problems, use kelp only once a day or less (long-term use is not recommended) and do not use if you have hyperthyroidism. Always take kelp capsules with water or a meal.

Do the shoulder stand. A yoga pose called the shoulder stand stimulates and massages the thyroid gland, explains Dr. Roberts. "It's one of the nicest ways to strengthen the mind-body connection." (See the illustration above.)

Go easy on foods that suppress thyroid function. Certain foods, such as cabbage, radishes, rutabagas, turnips, peaches, peanuts, soybeans, and spinach, can interfere with the production of thyroid hormones, especially when eaten raw. These foods, called goitrogens, won't cause a thyroid disorder but may aggravate an existing one. You don't need to avoid these foods altogether; simply don't eat a lot of them, says

Dr. Weil. On the other hand, if you have an *overactive* thyroid, eating more of these foods may help curb overproduction of thyroid hormone.

Turn to an herb. Bugleweed is a member of the mint family that's historically been used to support thyroid function, says Gayle Eversole, Ph.D., a nurse practitioner and professional member of the American Herbalists Guild in Granite Falls, Washington. It continues to be widely used in Europe as an herbal treatment for early-stage Graves' disease, often in combination with lemon balm. Preliminary studies in Germany suggest that bugleweed tincture can indeed reduce levels of thyroid hormone. The herb inhibits iodine absorption and reduces the amount of hormone produced by the thyroid gland.

Testosterone: It's Not Just Your Husband's Hormone

If hitting an unexpected speed bump with your car equates to the best sex you've had lately, you know your hormones are sending you a signal.

Nearly three out of four women suffer from some kind of sexual difficulty, whether it's decreased sex drive, vaginal dryness, or trouble reaching orgasm. Even if we don't have any severe sexual dysfunction, nearly all of us, according to one survey, have at least one sexual concern.

In the past, the best advice doctors usually offered to improve our sex lives—if we had the nerve to ask—ran from drinking a glass of wine to buying some lingerie. Most likely, they'd claim it was all in our heads.

And it's true that emotions and relationship issues are indeed a huge part of desire and sex. But researchers are discovering that, quite often, the problem lies in our hormones, which become more finicky as we age.

But getting older doesn't have to equate with making love less often. In one study, women over 65 had almost 10 percent more sex than women 39 to 50. Drug companies, inspired by men's reaction to the arousal drug Viagra, are discovering an equally enthusiastic, untapped market in women.

The good news is that the enormous amounts of research resulting from this quest provide numerous ways we can preserve our sexual function *without drugs* and knowledge we can use now to have better sex—*tonight*.

Stage One: Attraction

Perhaps there's no better way to explain the complex symphony of hormones involved in your love life than to provide a (sort of) real-life example. So curl up on the couch and pretend you're reading one of those steamy romance novels. . . .

While picking through some semi-bruised melons, your arm brushes up against something firm but furry. "Oh, excuse me," you say, turning just in time to bump heads with a salt-and-pepper-haired, blue-eyed, fellow melon fondler. You blush.

His eyes twinkle. "No problem," he smiles, handing you a cantaloupe. "This one's just right."

Your heart pounds, and you feel the blood rush to your face. "Thanks," you murmur, turning away to take a deep breath. *He's gorgeous!!* you think. Then, *He's probably taken.* You will yourself to forget him.

You fail.

Chalk up another victim to hormones. You're pumping out some serious pheromones—scentless hormones your salt-and-pepper stranger subconsciously receives and reacts to. Both men and women secrete pheromones in the skin oil around their nipples, armpits, and genitals. The brain senses them and alerts these pheromone-producing parts of the body to send their powerful signals of attraction back and forth.

They're particularly potent when we're most fertile, at ovulation. One study found that when men were exposed to the pheromones of ovulating women, their testosterone levels increased more than when they were exposed to pheromones of premenstrual or menstrual women. Our own libido-boosting testosterone levels also happen to be highest at ovulation—another way nature tries to get us together when it really counts.

Stage Two: Desire

Try as you might to forget him, you're a goner. You meet him again in the dairy aisle. As he leans over

WOMEN ASK WHY

Why doesn't my doctor talk to me about sexual issues?

Historically, medical doctors haven't had any answers for female sex questions. Plus, they're not trained on the topic in medical school and are often just as uncomfortable as anyone else talking about sex.

Women are repeatedly told their lagging sex drive is all in their heads or that it's something they must accept about aging. Often, doctors just blow them off or send them to therapists, which may or may not be appropriate. One solution is to get more sex education into medical school training, so physicians can start dealing with this proactively.

In the meantime, women can inform themselves. Look for information on the Web at sites like NEWSHE (Network for Excellence in Women's Sexual Health, www.newshe.com), which offers resources for women dealing with issues like lack of desire, arousal, lubrication, orgasm, and pain.

When you make a medical appointment, ask if your doctor has an e-mail address. Send her a list of questions, so she'll be prepared for your visit. Try to be as specific as possible: "Ever since I started having hot flashes, I notice I feel a bit drier—why is that?" or "My orgasms aren't as strong as they once were—what does that mean?" If you're uncomfortable just blurting these out, mention your recent anniversary or talk about your daughter's departure for college and how you'll be spending more time with your husband. Referring to your relationship might make it easier to transition into a discussion about sex.

Be firm about getting your needs addressed. You really don't have to take no for an answer. Some physicians are willing to help; they just may not know what to do. But the best ones are always willing to listen.

Expert consulted
Laura Berman, Ph.D.
Co-director of the Women's Sexual Health Clinic
Boston University Medical Center

to get some fat-free yogurt, you steal a glance, admiring the way his shorts show off his long, muscular legs and flat stomach. *Must play a lot of tennis*, you think to yourself. *He can win my "love" any time!* Without thinking, you giggle out loud. Salt-and-pepper looks up and grins.

"You're certainly enjoying your shopping today," he says. He glances at his watch. "Do you have anything that'll melt, or would you like to go for coffee next door? By the way, I'm Jay."

"Nope, nothing that will melt," you say, figuring you'll dump the ice cream on the way to the checkout counter. "I'd love to, Jay." Game, set, match!

By now, testosterone has arrived on the scene, triumphantly leading a full marching band of sex hormones and hormone-like neurotransmitters. Testosterone planted those fantasies in your brain, and it's probably making you tingle all over. Adrenaline is thumping the bass drum of your heart, and endorphins, nature's pleasure drugs, are reverberating through you like the crash of a cymbal.

Because you've decided he's worth a second glance, you're also producing the hormone oxytocin. Known as the touch-me hormone, oxytocin is released from the pituitary gland whenever we're close to the object of our affection, helping bond us to him. While oxytocin levels are simmering at a relatively low level right now, as soon as Jay puts his hand on your waist, they'll start a vigorous climb.

WOMAN TO WOMAN

She Had Testosterone Replacement Therapy

After Julia had her uterus and ovaries removed, her doctor brushed off her lack of desire, telling her, "It's all in your head." Fifteen years later, the New York resident discovered the truth: It was partly in her head, partly in her blood. With the successful addition of testosterone to her hormone replacement therapy—and a generous dose of couples therapy—Julia, now 69, and her husband have resumed a happy, healthy sex life.

It basically started about the time I had my uterus and ovaries removed, when I was 48. Because I'd had severe pain and bleeding from a prolapsed uterus and also had endometrial hyperplasia and a uterine cyst, my health improved dramatically after the surgery. But that's when my libido started to go.

When I went for a checkup soon thereafter, I told my doctor I wasn't as interested in sex and asked if it had anything to do with the hysterectomy. He said no and that normally women experience a gain in libido because of the freedom from pregnancy. He insinuated that it was "all in my head" and told me I'd get over it.

I believed him, mostly because it was hard to tell if my lack of desire was physical or emotional. My husband was going through his own midlife crisis at that time, and we became

Stage Three: Arousal

"I sure am glad you like melons," Jay says, pushing back a strand of your hair and looking deep into your eyes while the two of you stand outside your front door. Your last few dates have gotten progressively more romantic, and Jay has told you he loves you. Tonight may be The Night.

"I always was a sucker for a juicy piece of fruit," you joke, looking at your feet. *Invite him in!* testosterone screams.

very distant. Things dragged for years. My orgasms just disappeared.

I stayed with my gynecologist until he retired, assuming all along it was a relationship issue. About 6 years ago, my husband and I decided to seriously look at our relationship. We started seeing a couples therapist, and once we'd sorted out some of the major problems, she put us in touch with a psychiatric sex therapist. My husband was diagnosed with medical impotence and treated with drugs. Everything else was in place, but I still wasn't able to have an orgasm. That's when I realized it had to be physical.

My new doctor did a blood test and found my testosterone levels were nearly nonexistent. She put me on Winstrol to go along with the Premarin I was already taking. Very soon after I started the testosterone, I felt numerous physical changes: I was more interested in sex and able to have orgasms, but I also felt better, sharper. It was like I got a boost. I started working out more. There was a lot of emotional healing going on at the same time, but I definitely think the testosterone made a great difference. The two went hand in hand.

We're now very sexually active—we have sex at least once a week. It's really changed our marriage. The whole experience has confirmed my belief that any kind of physical problem also carries with it an emotional problem.

I can't wait much longer! You look up and give him a mischievous smile. "Speaking of, would you like to come in? I have some fresh honeydew."

Although you have only one-tenth the amount of testosterone Jay has, that doesn't mean you're only one-tenth as excited—far from it. Your adrenal glands and ovaries kick out half of your testosterone. The rest is produced by prehormones, like DHEA, that are converted to testosterone by your fat, skin, and muscle. About 1 percent of this testosterone is "free," however, the only kind that can actually influence your libido. But that 1 percent is busy chatting in your ear, sketching out scenarios, and building anticipation for what's to come.

Estrogen's also in the picture, priming you for takeoff, making sure that you're lubricated and that enough blood is being sent to your vagina. By keeping your vaginal tissues plump and filled with oxygen, estrogen helps you become easily engorged, exposing the maximum number of nerve endings so that you can really enjoy yourself.

Stage Four: Orgasm

It's never been like this before, you think, moving easily together with Jay. *I can't believe my luck!*

Again, send a silent thanks to your hormones. Testosterone maximizes your clitoral sensation and also renders your nipples tender and receptive to touch. Estrogen keeps your skin soft, inducing Jay to stroke it appreciatively, which, in turn, boosts your oxytocin levels even higher, making your skin even more sensitive in a win-win feedback loop that keeps circling higher. Suddenly, waves crash over you from all sides. With your orgasm, your oxytocin spikes to five times the level it reached during that first touch at the grocery store—and it stays high so you can enjoy cuddling when you collapse in the afterglow.

That is, until Jay falls asleep. He can't help it—he's drunk on oxytocin. Because you frequently touch your friends and acquaintances, you're accustomed to feeling this flush and are therefore less at its mercy. You also have more estrogen than Jay, a key factor in women's supe-

WOMEN ASK WHY

Why do men always want to have sex in the morning?

Men tend to have erections very easily in the morning because their levels of testosterone peak between 5:00 and 6:00 A.M. A lot of people misinterpret that to mean they're sexually excited, but that's not necessarily the truth. They may start to feel desire *because* they have an erection. Sometimes, men also have to go to the bathroom early in the morning. A full bladder can also be signaled by an erection, something researchers refer to as a "pee-on."

Because time is short in the morning, men may also look at a quickie as a way to start the day off on the right foot. Here's a secret: Many women like morning sex, too. Actually, women share this morning testosterone peak, as well as the evening testosterone dip, so morning sex could be an equal excitement opportunity.

Expert consulted
Janell Carroll, Ph.D.
Sex therapist and adjunct professor of psychology
University of Hartford
Connecticut

rior ability to use oxytocin on a day-to-day basis. So when Jay's hit with this onslaught, it really throws him for a loop! Well, at least it'll help you get a deep, restorative sleep. You'll need it—in the morning, both of your testosterone levels will hit their daily peaks.

When Your Sex Life Hits the Skids

Okay, so you know sex is great. But what if you haven't felt like having any lately? Or what if you realize that when you look at your hus-band these days, instead of scheming how to get him alone, you're only thinking that he needs to lose a few pounds and toss that shirt. When you were younger, it took only 10 to 15 seconds for you to get excited. After menopause, it can take 5 minutes, by which time you're usually asleep.

Again, blame hormones.

Libido and arousal are so reliant on our hormones' cooperation that when they're otherwise occupied, sex is often the first thing to go. The following are the five key times in your life when your sex hormones might go AWOL, say experts.

Pregnancy and breastfeeding. Moms are in for a bit of a dry spell. For as long as you breastfeed, your pituitary glands produce prolactin, a hormone that makes breastfeeding possible but that has a pronounced downer effect on your sex life by lowering levels of libido-raising hormones estrogen and testosterone.

Mild depression, anxiety, and hostility have also been associated with high levels of prolactin, and the link between low spirits and low libido is undeniable. In fact, decreased sexual desire is one of the symptoms of depression, says Sara-Jane Mize, Ph.D., assistant professor of psychology at the University of Minnesota Medical School in Minneapolis.

Stress. The first place stress hits is the adrenal glands, which produce a quarter of your body's testosterone, plus DHEA and other hormones that will eventually be converted into testosterone, says Deborah Moskowitz, N.D., managing physician at Transitions for Health, a company that provides natural products for women's health and hormone balance, in Portland, Oregon. When you're stressed, you produce more adrenaline and other corticosteroids, the hormones that help your body gear up for crises.

That wouldn't be such a big deal if you had only *fun* stress, such as roller-coaster rides. During this kind of stress, the sympathetic nervous system gets a rush that can help put you in the mood, says Cindy Meston, Ph.D., sex researcher and assistant professor of psychology at the University of Texas at Austin. But our lives are *packed* with minor crises. Some alternative medical experts speculate that this constant overload can cause the adrenals to slow down, sending your body into "adrenopause." That can lead to extreme levels of fatigue and severely limit hormone function, including the hormones that contribute to sex drive, says Dr. Moskowitz.

So why do men typically want to have sex no matter how stressed they are? Their adrenals produce only 5 percent of their testosterone, so they're not nearly as dependent on the glands for their sex drive.

Menopause and hysterectomy. Along with hot flashes and sleepless nights, menopause can wreak havoc on your sex life. After your ovaries stop producing estrogen, what little you have left comes from the conversion of the increasingly limited supply of DHEA and testosterone from the adrenals. With an ovarian hysterectomy, the effects are even

DO YOU HAVE SEXUAL PROBLEMS?

Kevin Billups, M.D., a urologist specializing in female sexual dysfunction in St. Paul, Minnesota, created this simple quiz for women who suspect they have female sexual arousal disorder.

Ask yourself the following questions.

1. Has the sensation in your vagina decreased?
   Yes   No   Unsure

2. When you're being sexually stimulated, has your amount of vaginal lubrication decreased?
   Yes   No   Unsure

3. Is vaginal penetration more painful now?
   Yes   No   Unsure

4. Is it more difficult to have an orgasm through intercourse?
   Yes   No   Unsure

5. Has it become more difficult to have an orgasm from stimulating your clitoris?
   Yes   No   Unsure

6. Has the feeling in your clitoris during stimulation or intercourse decreased?
   Yes   No   Unsure

7. Has the feeling in your vagina during stimulation or intercourse decreased?
   Yes   No   Unsure

8. Has your desire for sex and intercourse decreased?
   Yes   No   Unsure

9. Has your overall sexual satisfaction during intercourse or stimulation decreased?
   Yes   No   Unsure

If you answered yes to any of the questions above, it's time to talk to your doctor about your decreased satisfaction with your sex life.

more dramatic: Your testosterone levels are cut in half overnight.

Declining estrogen minimizes sensation in the labia, interferes with lubrication, and makes the tissues in the vagina very delicate and prone to bleeding—certainly not a recipe for hot sex. A study conducted at Boston University Medical Center found that 67 percent of menopausal women experienced low arousal and pain during sex—and a whopping 92 percent had trouble reaching orgasm.

The impact is also psychological. "When you have estrogen on board, your skin is soft and supple, the breasts are fuller," says Barbara Bartlik, M.D., assistant professor of psychiatry at the Weill Medical College of Cornell University in New York City. "When the estrogen goes, all that changes, so the way you feel about your attractiveness can change."

Not all is lost. Hormone replacement therapy can help. Besides keeping your vaginal tissues healthy and well-lubricated, supplemental estrogen may help arousal by activating oxytocin and increasing the body's production of the neurotransmitter nitric oxide, in much the same way Viagra does (see "Viagra and Other Sex Drugs for Women" on page 166).

Hormone Replacement and Birth Control Pills

Although estrogen replacement can help ease certain sex-related symptoms, it can sometimes rebound. When estrogen is introduced to the body from the outside, it may "swamp out" all other sex hormones—including testosterone—because it raises the level of a protein called sex hormone binding globulin (SHBG), says Dr. Moskowitz. If SHBG binds to sex hormones, whether estrogen or testosterone, it makes them less active. An internal battle of the sexes com-

mences as testosterone tries to limit SHBG production in the liver, and the supplemental estrogen fights back by raising it. Estrogen wins out, because SHBG attaches to testosterone three times more readily and strongly than to estrogen.

So while the supplemental estrogen is priming your body, the lack of testosterone is sending any interest in making love out the window. Switching to a hormone replacement medication that includes testosterone, like Estratest, might help restore your desire, says Dr. Bartlik.

Synthetic progesterone (called progestin), often part of hormone replacement therapy and birth control pills, can also have negative effects. Naturally occurring progesterone helps make testosterone and estrogen, so maintaining certain levels is necessary. But the synthetic progestins in birth control pills and HRT trick the body into thinking it's pregnant and may also dampen the sex drive and interfere with lubrication.

Boost Your Sex Hormones Naturally

We can boost our hormones—or at least outsmart them—with exercise, nutrition, herbs, good habits, and, yes, sex. Here are some things to try.

Blast testosterone-hogging fat. Excessive body fat can convert testosterone into estrogen, so improving your muscle-to-fat ratio through exercise may improve your libido, says Dr. Bartlik. Some doctors also believe that exercise boosts levels of DHEA, a precursor of testosterone. Aerobic exercise itself actually wakes up your nerves and primes your sympathetic nervous system for sex, says Dr. Meston. Exercise also improves your cardiovascular system and increases blood flow, a key part of arousal and orgasm.

Yoga, a more sedate exercise, may also help, says Dr. Moskowitz. She recommends Ashtanga, a variety of yoga involving poses that clench and tone the Kegel muscles, driving blood flow back into the pelvic region. Or you could just clench your pelvic muscles several times a day and right before sex to stimulate those nerves and make your blood flow more easily and quickly, she says.

Break bad habits. Quitting smoking may dramatically improve your sex life, says Dr. Moskowitz. When you smoke, you decrease the oxygen flow throughout your body, and we've already covered the benefits of a healthy blood supply to your vagina. Smoking also depletes estrogen stores in the body, causing female smokers to enter menopause several years before nonsmokers. Smokers also get less vaginal lubrication. And because nicotine concentrates itself in the cervical tissues, researchers believe it damages the DNA of cervical cells and may contribute to the development of cervical cancer.

Communicate and reconnect. Ask yourself this: "If I had a week away from my job, kids, and responsibilities and I could go anywhere in the world with my husband, would I feel like having sex?"

"If the answer is yes, then your problem is not physical," says Janell Carroll, Ph.D., sex therapist and adjunct professor of psychology at the

THE POSTAGE STAMP TEST

For many years, neither snow nor rain nor heat nor gloom of night could stay your partner from swift and passionate completion in the bedroom. But lately, your postman is no longer ringing twice, and you're wondering how to get him back to his appointed rounds.

Look no further than the U.S. Postal Service.

Researchers have developed a way to use stamps to determine whether men have physical or psychological impotence. It works like this: A strip of stamps is wrapped around a man's penis before bed. If the stamps are broken in the morning, it means he's able to have a nighttime erection. And that means his impotence may be psychological, rather than physical, since men normally experience several erections during the course of the night.

Physical impotence has many possible sources. As men age, they may develop diabetes or heart disease, or they may have excess fat or bad smoking habits—all of which can interfere with their ability to become aroused. When physically healthy men go into REM sleep, they can experience up to four erections a night. These erections have nothing to do with arousal or desire—they're simply a routine physical function.

A study conducted at the Jefferson Sexual Function Center of Jefferson Medical College in Philadelphia found the stamp test to be 83 percent effective in determining if a man had a physical source of impotence.

To try it at home, take a roll of stamps and wrap a strip around the base of your partner's penis before he goes to bed. If the strip isn't broken in the morning, have him see a urologist. If it is broken, this may be a great way to open a discussion about sex and how it's changed for both of you. Gently reassure him that you're in this together, advises sex therapist Janell Carroll, Ph.D., of the University of Hartford in Connecticut, who conducted the stamp study. But don't discount the effect his impotence has on your own libido—her research found that 41 percent of the sexual partners of men with impotence blamed themselves.

University of Hartford in Connecticut. Remember, your marriage is the foundation of your family, and you need to honor it accordingly, says Dr. Carroll. Farm the kids off to their friends' houses for a sleepover, but try something new—instead of going out for dinner, stay home. Prepare a meal together, light some candles, use the good china—then make love on the dining room table (or the couch or stairs or anywhere *except* the bedroom).

Eat right. In addition to all the usual recommendations, make sure you're getting your fair share of the following.

- *Soy.* Just as soy isoflavones have the potential to help manage various symptoms of menopause, these phytoestrogens may help lessen the severity of your hot flashes. Intense hot flashes can make you feel irritable and prevent a restful night's sleep—both factors that could impact a good sex life, says Dr. Moskowitz. She recommends 60 milligrams a day of soy protein, found in a tofu burger with soy cheese, a large glass of soy milk, or a half-cup of roasted soy nuts.

- *B vitamins.* These vitamins are heavily involved in the production of cell energy and can help guarantee the highest level of testosterone production and release by supporting the adrenal glands. Those glands, as you recall, are responsible for a quarter of all testosterone production. Dr. Moskowitz suggests one complete B-complex supplement (all the different B vitamins together) per day.

- *Fish.* Estrogen and testosterone are derived from cholesterol, so eating a little animal protein could help preserve your sex drive, says Dr. Moskowitz. When you get this protein from fish, you stand to reap even larger dividends: Studies have linked fish consumption with lower rates of cardiovas-cular disease and heart attacks. DHA, an omega-3 fatty acid found in cold-water fish like salmon, tuna, and mackerel, may also prevent depression and keep up your spirits—a key factor in a healthy and happy sex life. Just three servings of fish a week may provide these benefits.

Have a drink or two. But keep it at that. Although alcohol can lower inhibitions and may be perceived as helping your sex drive, more than two drinks may actually interfere with libido, says Dr. Moskowitz. Finnish researchers found that one or two drinks may boost testosterone, but more than that on a long-term basis can minimize its power by damaging nerves and interfering with your body's ability to become aroused.

Try herbs. These are especially good choices.

- *Astralagus.* It's an adaptogen, an herb that helps the body adapt to physical and emotional stress. By helping you manage stress better, it can relieve some of the toll on the adrenals, which can help keep testosterone and other hormones in correct balance. Dr. Moskowitz usually recommends 100 to 500 milligrams a day in capsule form, and it can be used long term.

- *Motherwort.* "This herb has a lot of hormone-balancing and phytoestrogen effects," says Dr. Moskowitz. "Historically, it's been used for low libido after menopause." She recommends 100 to 200 milligrams a day in capsule form.

- *Ginkgo.* It's widely used for memory problems because it increases blood flow in the brain, but it also helps with the pelvic area, says Dr. Moskowitz. "When you increase blood flow to that area, you're increasing the health of the tissues, muscles, and nerves." She recommends 60 to 120 milligrams, standardized to 24 percent glycosides, per day.

Try everything—but sex. Even if you're not interested in intercourse just now, touching and hugging your partner can boost oxytocin and other hormones associated with arousal and orgasm, says Dr. Bartlik. If you take it to the level of massage, you'll encourage the release of endorphins to help stir things up, says Larry Feldman, M.D., director of the Pain and Stress Rehabilitation Center in New Castle, Delaware.

Fantasize. "Sexual fantasy is actually a great way to build desire," says David Glass, Ph.D., a clinical psychologist and sex therapist in Arlington, Virginia.

Follow the sex pyramid. Dr. Mize and her colleagues use a "Pyramid of Sexuality" to describe some of the behaviors involved with sex that may be neglected as a relationship becomes more routine.

Dr. Mize stresses that the behaviors at the base might be the most comfortable for some couples to engage in and can provide the basis for progression to the top of the pyramid.

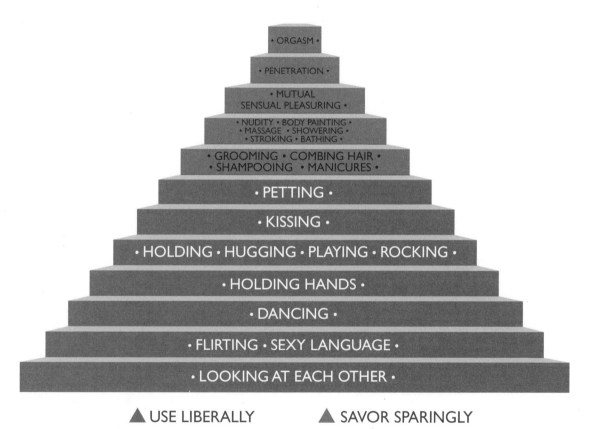

▲ USE LIBERALLY   ▲ SAVOR SPARINGLY

To use this sex pyramid, sample the bottom tiers daily, savor top tiers happily, and combine all liberally for a full and healthy sex life!

Fight or Flight: The Stress Hormones

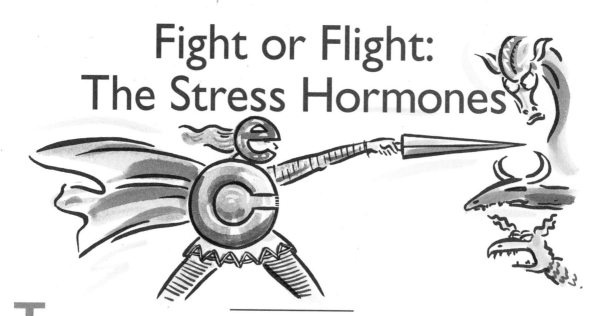

Think back to that last traffic jam or job deadline. Remember how your heart raced, your palms sweated, your muscles tensed? You blamed it on the accident up ahead or on an unreasonable boss. Instead, blame it on hormones.

Yup, your reactions to stress are controlled by chemicals with such tongue-twisting names as cortisol, adrenaline (also called epinephrine), and noradrenaline (also called norepinephrine).

Although you can't really prevent hormones from kicking in, you can learn to control how you respond to stress and moderate those hormonal reactions. Proven techniques range from deep breathing and yoga to journaling, herbs, and vitamins.

This Thing Called Stress

The term was coined back in the 1930s by researcher Hans Selye, M.D. In his lab work with rats, Dr. Selye learned that those accidentally dropped during experiments suffered more ulcers than rats that had not been dropped. He also noticed that the dropped rats were more likely to have high blood pressure, tense muscles,

dilated pupils, and hormonal changes than the other rats.

Over the years, we've learned that humans are not so different from those stressed-out rats. But it is only in recent years that researchers have honed in on a greater understanding of how hormones relate to stress and how that hormonal response can sometimes go awry, leaving us chronically frayed and at risk for other health problems.

We've also learned about the genetic components of stress—again, hormonally related. For instance, studies show that depressed women who are pregnant pass along high levels of the stress hormone cortisol to their fetuses, says Maria Hernandez-Reif, Ph.D., director of research at the Touch Research Institute at the University of Miami School of Medicine. That makes the baby more susceptible to stress-related problems through development.

Even how we're born can affect our lifelong ability to handle stress. In one study, babies born by assisted delivery (such as forceps or emergency cesarean) had higher levels of cortisol than those delivered by elective cesarean section. And research with rat pups—which scientists say is applicable to humans—shows that babies neglected in their first week of life have higher levels of stress hormones, which appear to last into adulthood.

Stress is not all bad, however. We actually need *some* stress. It keeps us going from day to day, motivating and invigorating us to participate in hobbies, sports, and friendships or to meet job deadlines and even keep our homes and yards tidy. Heck, some women clean only when they *are* stressed!

Of course, what is stressful to one woman may be just a yawn to another. It's how we *perceive* an event that precipitates the stress reaction and determines the magnitude of our hormonal response. For instance, one woman may thrive on rock climbing and skydiving, while another finds a 20-mile drive on the freeway terrifying.

There's even a book titled *Stressed Is Desserts Spelled Backwards*!

But when the baby's screaming, the rice is boiling over, and company is arriving from out of town the next day, we probably aren't going to compare stress with a tasty slice of Key lime pie. We're more likely to feel as if we're wading waist deep through a river of mud.

Again, blame hormones.

Our Brains on Stress

No matter what the stressor—a traffic jam, running late for an appointment, laundry that's piling up, grief over the loss of a loved one, or a life-endangering threat such as a mugging—our basic physiological response is the same. A signal goes out to the grape-sized control center deep inside our brains called the hypothalamus. Think of it as the 911 command center of stress.

Only instead of dispatching the police to your home, it dispatches CRH (corticotropin re-

---

ARE YOU SICK—OR STRESSED?

Your mother just left after a 2-week visit, you just sent the kids back to school, and you got your car back after that fender bender. Life is finally returning to normal when your throat starts to feel scratchy and you begin sneezing. Like clockwork, you can count on stress to affect you physically, from colds and flu to cancer and heart disease.

While acute, short-lived stress—such as sitting in traffic or waiting at the bank drive-thru when you're in a hurry—may stimulate immunity, studies show chronic stress dampens it. Again, blame that pesky hormone cortisol, which destroys immune cells when it's chronically elevated, says Maria Hernandez-Reif, Ph.D., director of research at the Touch Research Institute at the University of Miami School of Medicine.

Cortisol damages your body's natural killer cells, which search out and destroy tumors and help fight viruses and infections, Dr. Hernandez-Reif says. Women with breast cancer, for example, have high levels of cortisol.

In one study at Ohio State University, researchers found that breast-cancer patients with high anxiety experienced a 20 to 30 percent decrease in their natural killer cells' ability to fend off infection and cancer.

But you don't need to have cancer to stress your immune system. Even arguments with family or friends can do it, according to studies by Janice Kiecolt-Glaser, Ph.D., director of health psychiatry at Ohio State in Columbus.

If you know you're headed for a difficult time, practicing such proven stress-reducing techniques as exercise, yoga, deep breathing, and guided imagery may help you prepare.

leasing hormone), setting off a cascade of action. The CRH zips down a stalk-like connection to the pituitary gland at the base of the brain, which releases the chemical ACTH (adrenocorticotrophic hormone). Then ACTH fires up the production of cortisol—the main stress hormone—in the adrenals, a pair of small, triangular glands that sit atop the kidneys, and the cortisol courses through the bloodstream.

Although cortisol has gotten a bad rap in the stress lexicon, it's actually not the enemy. It plays a valuable role when we're physically or emotionally stressed, helping regulate blood pressure, balance insulin as it breaks down sugar for energy, prevent inflammation if we're wounded, and fight infection. It also initially sharpens our attention, so we're ready to act.

In the meantime, our adrenal glands also spurt out the hormones adrenaline and noradrenaline, which prepare us to flee if we're facing a threat. Our hearts race, our breathing quickens, our blood pressures climb, our muscles tense, and our blood sugar is turned into energy. We may feel sweaty or as though our hair is standing on end.

Almost 70 years ago, researcher Walter Cannon, M.D., called the experience "the fight-or-flight" response—the same rush of hormones that signaled our ancient ancestors to either do battle or run when facing danger. Think lions, tigers, and bears.

Even though we're not facing those kinds of stressors today, our brains still work the same, says Ruth E. Quillian, Ph.D., a health psychologist at Duke University's Center for Living in Durham, North Carolina.

Once the threat has passed, adrenaline, noradrenaline, and cortisol drop off as the parasympathetic nervous system takes over, triggering hormones like oxytocin to soothe and calm us, returning our bodies to balance—what scientists call homeostasis.

If we're under daily or extreme stress, though, the cortisol never stops flowing. Even good stress, such as marrying or buying a home, can keep cortisol running like water through an open faucet, though researchers still don't know why.

The more constant the release of cortisol, the more depleted the adrenals become, says Rebecca Wynsome, N.D., medical director of Water's Edge Natural Health Services and a naturopathic physician in Seattle. That's the cause of fatigue for many women, she says.

In her patients with chronic fatigue syndrome, for instance, "their cortisol is often too low," Dr. Wynsome says. In other words, the vicious stress cycle has left them without enough of the hormone to battle even the normal stressors they encounter every day.

Such chronic stress may also deplete our supply of adrenaline, leaving us feeling exhausted and unable to meet daily demands. This adrenal dysfunction may contribute to foggy thinking, sleep problems, low blood sugar, infections, headaches, depression, forgetfulness—and even a hankering for sweets.

Overproduction of cortisol, however, is the apparent culprit in many stress-induced maladies, says John Newcomer, M.D., associate professor of psychiatry at Washington University School of Medicine in St. Louis.

Researchers made the cortisol connection after studying patients with Cushing's syndrome, a rare disease in which people pump out too much of the hormone. Symptoms include diabetes, muscle weakness, skin disorders, osteoporosis, high blood pressure, anxiety, and depression—which, oddly enough, are all also related to stress.

Also, cortisol-related drugs such as prednisone (typically given to reduce the inflammation of arthritis or asthma) sometimes cause serious, stress-related psychiatric side effects, including depression, weight gain, and forgetfulness, in as many as 20 percent of patients. Minor effects such as subtle memory loss and irritability occur in up to 90 percent of patients, says Owen M. Wolkowitz, M.D., professor of psychiatry at the University of California at San Francisco's medical center, who has extensively studied stress hormones.

You're Not Losing Your Mind—You're Just Stressed

How many times in the past week have you walked into a room and wondered why you were there? Tried to introduce a friend and realized that you'd forgotten her name? Put the milk in the kitchen cabinet and the cereal in the refrigerator?

You're not crazy. You're just stressed.

Several researchers have shown that high cortisol can make it difficult to learn or memorize new information.

In one study at the University of Washington in St. Louis, 51 participants, half of them women, took high-dose cortisol capsules twice daily—amounts comparable to what we might release if we were having abdominal surgery or witnessing a tragedy. The subjects fared worse on memory tests after 4 days than those who received low-dose capsules or a placebo (inactive pill).

BLAME IT ON HORMONES
Facial Hair

You shave your legs, your underarms, even your bikini area. But your face?

Yup. About 20 million American women try to conceal or remove facial hair at least once a week.

"There are some women out there shaving two times a day," says Amy McMichael, M.D., assistant professor of dermatology at Wake Forest University in Winston-Salem, North Carolina. She helped develop a cream that slows the growth of facial hair in women.

As we age and our estrogen levels drop, problems with facial hair may get worse, she says.

For up to 90 percent of women with facial hair, there is no underlying problem. But if you experience any sudden change in hair growth—especially in typically male areas such as the cheeks—see a doctor. In about 10 percent of women, such changes could be caused by a tumor, polycystic ovarian disease, or a benign condition called hirsutism, in which hair grows fast, thick, and on the cheeks, chin, forehead, and chest.

There is no cure for hirsutism. But the cream Dr. McMichael helped test, called Vaniqa (eflornithine HCl), slows hair growth—no matter the cause.

Oral contraceptives, hormone replacement therapy, and a prescription drug called spironolactone (which reduces the male hormones floating around our bodies) may also help reduce unwanted hair. Keep your boyfriend or husband away from Vaniqa, though. It hasn't been found safe for men, who might be tempted to try it as an alternative to daily shaving.

Of course, you can always follow the tried and true: shaving, waxing, depilatories, electrolysis, and the new laser therapies. One home remedy is "sugaring." Sugar and water are boiled together, as when making candy, until they reach a taffy-like consistency. Once cool, the mixture is applied to the skin and then pulled off as you would wax. You can refrigerate the mixture and reuse it (hand-kneading under warm water first).

Interestingly, those taking high levels of cortisol didn't *feel* stressed out. They weren't anxious, nor were they aware they scored lower on the tests. Other researchers have shown memory plummets within an hour after administering supplemental cortisol, says Dr. Newcomer.

Once stress retreats and cortisol levels fall, however, these effects are reversed. In the St. Louis study, for instance, the participants' learning and recall capacities returned in about a week.

Researchers speculate that these and other findings may explain why we often become forgetful when we take a test, interview for a job, or give courtroom testimony.

Studies show that cortisol may cause other memory problems as we age. Too much of the hormone over time might contribute to a decrease in the hippocampus, the part of the brain that helps us remember people, places, and events. Some researchers speculate there may even be a connection between stress and amnesia or Alzheimer's disease.

Your Mood on Stress Hormones

The shrinking hippocampus may also be involved in the link between stress hormones and depression.

For instance, some research shows that long-term depression is associated with a smaller hippocampus and elevated cortisol. And women who are depressed often have higher levels of cortisol than their nondepressed counterparts.

The Amazing Properties of Oxytocin

You know the basics of "fight or flight": From primitive times, we've reacted to physical or emotional threat with anger and aggression—or with a hasty retreat.

Groundbreaking work by researchers at the University of California at Los Angeles is now turning fight or flight on its wing. For women, at least.

It seems that rather than responding in a fight-or-flight fashion when threatened, fearful, or stressed, women may be more inclined to "tend or befriend." We're more likely to protect and nurture our young and turn to family and friends for solace, says Laura Cousino Klein, Ph.D., one of six researchers to contribute to the theory.

It never made sense from an evolutionary standpoint for women to fight or flee, says Dr. Klein, now an assistant professor of behavioral health at Pennsylvania State University in University Park. It's a rare female of any species who would leave her babies to fend for themselves. It's more likely that we'd protect them, bonding with other females in the process.

The notion of tend or befriend first occurred to Dr. Klein in 1998, after she and fellow UCLA researcher Shelley E. Taylor, Ph.D., listened to a presentation on depression, immunity, and serotonin, which mentioned rats and the fight-or-flight response.

Dr. Taylor, a professor of psychology, told Dr. Klein she didn't typically see that kind of reaction from women under stress. Neither had Dr. Klein. The lightbulb went on, and when the researchers delved deeper into studies over the past 15 years, they found that only about 4,000 out of 15,000 animal and human subjects in stress-related experiments had been female.

Moreover, the females generally responded differently than the males. For example, mothers whose rat pups were removed from their care tended to soothe the babies by

Dr. Wolkowitz also is looking at the role of the hormone DHEA, or dehydroepiandrosterone, in depression. It appears that the higher the DHEA levels, the lower the likelihood of

grooming and nursing them when they were reunited. And female primates would group together to fend off aggressive males and protect their young. Males tended to be more angry and aggressive when threatened, the studies showed. They were also more likely to flee or disengage—not unlike Dad after a tough day at work.

The reason, Dr. Taylor suggests, may be the hormone oxytocin, typically released during childbirth and breastfeeding. Both men and women produce it, but we churn out more. And in terms of research, it had been mostly forgotten.

Oxytocin, however, is a known mood regulator that's also released when we're stressed, Dr. Klein says. In fact, studies show oxytocin decreases anxiety and depression and promotes social bonding. So after a hard day's work, for example, women are more likely to talk with the kids, while men may need time to decompress.

So, when we're stressed—say, cut off in traffic—we still get that quick burst of epinephrine and norepinephrine; cortisol still hastens onto the scene. But then comes oxytocin, which hangs around just long enough to soothe and settle us—and send us seeking someone to talk to.

The female hormone estrogen enhances oxytocin's role and the tend-or-befriend response in women, while the male hormone testosterone appears to enhance the fight-or-flight reaction in men, says Dr. Klein.

That doesn't mean women never become angry or aggressive, of course, or that men never befriend or tend.

But the theory might lead to a better understanding between the sexes. (Think about John Gray's 1992 book *Men Are from Mars, Women Are from Venus*, in which Gray suggests that men solve problems in solitude, while women prefer to talk—and talk and talk and talk.)

Says Dr. Klein, "For a long time, we haven't known why that might be. Oxytocin could be part of the answer."

Neurotransmitters (nerve chemicals) such as serotonin and dopamine also boost mood. That ability is the basis for prescription antidepressants such as Prozac, Zoloft, Paxil, and Wellbutrin. Researchers may one day better understand how these neurotransmitters (which can also act as hormones) and hormones work together.

Am I Actually Hungry for That Chocolate Cake?

Why is it that the refrigerator or the cookie jar is often the first thing we turn to when we're stressed? Again, blame it on hormones.

One of cortisol's roles is to help our bodies refuel after the energy-depleting effects of that fender bender, that fight with our boss, or other stressors. Unrelenting stress, notes Pamela Peeke, M.D., in her book, *Fight Fat after Forty*, may result in a "raging appetite" and fat that settles around our waists and bellies.

In one Yale University study, 59 women were exposed to stressors—speech giving, math tests, puzzles—over 3 days. After each session, the women were able to eat as much as they wanted from baskets of chocolate granola bars, potato chips, rice cakes, and pretzels.

The women whose cortisol levels rose in response to the stressors were more likely to reach for sweet snacks. The results suggest that high levels of cortisol may lead to weight gain and related health problems, such as diabetes, heart disease, and stroke, says study researcher Elissa Epel, Ph.D., now a

depression. DHEA does not actually lower levels of cortisol or its production; rather, it may make certain effects of cortisol more intense.

researcher in health psychology at the University of California at San Francisco.

What's more, high cortisol makes insulin less effective, Dr. Epel says. So while you're bingeing on sweets after feeling stressed—and raising your blood sugar accordingly—your pancreas is pumping out more and more insulin in an effort to move that sugar into your cells. If you're feeling stressed, cortisol tells your cells to ignore the insulin, leaving the glucose in your bloodstream. Also, all that insulin promotes fat storage, which means you might pack on a few extra pounds.

The researchers suggested that having high cortisol, or stress, leads not only to weight gain but also to fat around the midsection. Such fat is linked to psychological vulnerabilities such as depression and anxiety and to physical illnesses such as diabetes and heart disease.

> ### WOMAN TO WOMAN
> #### *Yoga Was Her Answer*
>
> Abbie Korman, 43, of Virginia Beach, Virginia, lived life in the fast lane after graduating from college and landing a job at a Washington, D.C., television station. To keep up, she smoked cigarettes and gulped Maalox straight from the bottle. Then she turned to yoga. That was nearly two decades ago. Today, although Abbie no longer works in TV, smokes, or swigs antacids, she still practices yoga. This is her story.
>
> Not long after graduating from college, I began working as a talk show producer at a Washington television station. Talk about stress!
>
> There were some pluses to the job, though. For one, I produced several segments on health topics. After a program about yoga—how the breathing, stretching, and positioning could help us center ourselves and find calm—I spotted a flier for a class and signed up.
>
> I'd been a swimmer for a long time. That helped me burn energy and destress. But with yoga, I felt so relaxed. Although I didn't feel noticeably less stressed at work, the class became my timeout: I could focus on nothing but the precision of the movements.
>
> I continued the classes twice a week for a couple of years

Turning the Tables on Stress

Breathe deeply and you're on your way toward more relaxed living.

In his seminal book *The Relaxation Response*, Herbert H. Benson, M.D., laid the groundwork for much of what we know today about reducing stress and the hormones that accompany it.

Here's how it works: Find a quiet spot and a comfortable environment. Repeat a word or phrase while gently pushing away everyday thoughts and returning to your word. Try to find a word you feel good about, such as snow, rain, peace, calm.

Close your eyes and relax your muscles, from your neck down to your toes. Breathe slowly as you focus on your word and exhale. If other thoughts intrude, simply return to your word and your breathing. Take a few seconds before opening your eyes and getting back to your reality, advises Dr. Benson. Do this once or twice a week for about 20 minutes at a time.

Over the years, numerous studies in medical journals have shown that this method—and various versions of it—counteracts our fight-or-flight response and sends stress hormones such as epinephrine packing. It also lowers cortisol and raises DHEA.

but eventually drifted away because of my busy schedule. I was still swimming and occasionally worked out at a gym. Then, during one of my weight training workouts, I herniated two disks in my back. My doctor said I needed surgery. Before I consented to the operation, however, I went back to yoga to see if it might help.

Incredibly, it did. It reduced the pain in my back, not to mention my stress. I never did have the surgery—and I've practiced yoga ever since.

My husband, Rob, and I moved to Virginia Beach in 1986, and in 1991, I gave birth to my first child, Adam.

I wasn't working outside the home, but the stress of being a new mom was great. So one day, I treated myself to a massage. As it turned out, the massage therapist also was a yoga instructor. She suggested I try her classes, which I did. It was so relaxing!

Now, Rob and I have a second son, Michael, 6. I attend a yoga class almost every Saturday and practice it at home some mornings too. It helps keep me centered and better able to keep up with the demands of two young boys, a husband, and a home.

I've also become more aware of myself—both emotionally and physically—through yoga. And I'm able to let go of some of the stress that can get in the way of living fully.

In one study of 33 women ages 44 to 66, conducted at Harvard Medical School's Mind/Body Institute, which Dr. Benson heads, researchers showed that practicing the relaxation response daily over 10 weeks reduced hot flashes, tension, anxiety, and depression.

There are numerous other ways to elicit the relaxation response, experts say, including the following.

Yoga. The ancient practice of postures, gentle stretching, and focused breathing has been shown to lower stress hormones and improve the sense of well-being. A 3-month study of yoga training at Hanover Medical University in Germany showed decreases in adrenaline, noradrenaline, and cortisol among those who practiced it daily.

Many gyms and recreation centers offer classes in yoga, but there are some simple practices you can use in your own living room, such as the position called *savasana*.

Lie on your back on a mat, keeping your ankles about 18 inches apart and letting your feet fall outward. With palms upward, rest your arms about 6 inches from your body. Close your eyes and focus on your breathing—breathe slowly and deeply. Your belly should rise when you inhale and fall when you exhale. Notice the tension in your body and let it go, from muscle to muscle.

Qigong. This method of incorporating gentle exercise, breathing, and meditation with tai chi, a Japanese system of exercise, also elicits the relaxation response. Because both qigong and tai chi involve a series of precise movements, the methods are best learned with an instructor. Many gyms and recreation centers now offer classes in both.

For more information on qigong, visit the Web site of the East West Academy of Healing Arts in San Francisco at www.eastwestqi.com. To learn more about classes in tai chi, call the Taoist Tai Chi Society of the USA in Tallahassee, Florida, at (850) 224-5438 or go to the International Taoist Tai Chi Society's Web site at www.taoist.org.

Breath focus. Simply breathe normally, but pay attention to how your breath feels—in and out. Next, breathe deeply, slowly—in through your nose and all the way down to your belly. Let your belly poof up. Now, let out the breath through your mouth. Alternate between the normal breath and the belly breath several times. Notice how you feel. Take another 10 minutes and imagine peace and calm flowing in with each breath. Be aware of breathing out anxiety or stress.

Progressive muscle relaxation. Instead of simply breathing deeply to relax, tense and relax each muscle as you slowly inhale and exhale. Try this one lying down. Begin with your forehead, tightening the muscles to a count of five, then releasing them. Move down your body from your eyes, jaw, and neck to your chest, shoulders, arms, and hands. Then go on to your legs and feet. At each point, tighten your muscles to a count of five and release.

Guided imagery. With this technique, you use your mind to transport yourself to a calming place. Find a quiet, comfortable spot. Close your eyes and simply let your mind wander to a favorite place or experience. Drift to a placid lakeside, a deserted beach, or a wooded mountaintop. "Imagine yourself being there," says Angela Stroup, R.N., a certified hypnotherapist and assistant professor of family and community medicine at Eastern Virginia Medical School in Norfolk. See the brilliant yellows and reds, hear gently rippling waves, smell the freshly cut lawn, or feel the sand between your toes. Become absorbed in the experience.

Move Out of Stress

Vigorous exercise, such as running, fast walking, or bicycling, releases endorphins, hormones shown to dull pain and create a mild euphoria.

In one study of 12 healthy men and women at the University of North Carolina–Greensboro, for example, participants showed higher levels of endorphins after only 20 minutes of intense cycling on stationary bikes.

We don't need to pedal away on a stationary cycle or run a marathon to benefit, says Dixie Stanforth, a certified exercise professional at the University of Texas at Austin. Walk around the block, bounce a basketball, hit a tennis ball against a wall, or even toy with one of those little paddle balls with the elastic string, the kind we had when we were 6. Or simply rock in a rocking chair. Anything rhythmical is beneficial, Stanforth says. "You don't want the exercise to become the stressor."

Laugh a Little

Studies have long shown that humor and mirthful laughter can lower levels of adrenaline and cortisol. In one study at Stanford University, several minutes of intense laughter produced physiological results, such as increased heart rate, comparable to exercising aerobically for 15 minutes on a stationary cycle or a rowing machine. And researchers at Loma Linda University in California found that laughter not only lowered stress hormones but also raised natural killer cells that help the body fight infection.

Even just talking to yourself may help lower stress hormones and protect you from depression and illness.

Psychologists call it "cognitive behavioral therapy"—reframing your thinking from negative to positive. For example, when the car won't start in the morning and you're late for work, you could assume the whole day—maybe even the week—will go badly. That catastrophic thinking is likely to raise your cortisol levels and leave you feeling stressed most of the day. Yet, realistically, it isn't likely to happen. If you focus on fixing the problem—finding another ride, taking the day off, calling a taxi—without exaggerating the outcome, you'll be less likely to feel stressed.

Write It Down

One of the best ways to destress is to explore your thoughts and yourself through writing or journaling.

At the University of Texas, James W. Pennebaker, Ph.D., a psychologist and author of *Opening Up*, has completed about a dozen studies showing that women who spend 20 minutes a day for 4 days or so writing about their most painful or stressful experiences feel better psychologically and physically. Some become less anxious and less depressed. Others show improvements in symptoms of asthma and arthritis.

"Most recently, we found drops in blood pressure and salivary cortisol among employees of a large organization who were randomly assigned to write about emotional topics," Dr. Pennebaker says.

How to journal? Andrew Weil, M.D., director of the integrative medicine program and clinical professor of internal medicine at the University of Arizona College of Medicine in Tucson, suggests his patients write about their feelings for 15 to 20 minutes a day. Before each session, try quieting your mind by meditating or deep breathing. Put a date on your writing, so you can follow changes or patterns.

Write quickly and don't go back to make "corrections." Above all, tell yourself the truth! And keep your journal in a private place. If you don't like writing, Dr. Weil suggests a "visual" journal. Simply draw in a sketchbook, using crayons or colored pencils.

Massage Away Stress

Of course, lying in a darkened room and letting someone smooth scented oil over your body and gently knead your muscles is going to feel good. We know that intuitively, but it's always nice to know that researchers are out proving it scientifically.

In one study of 50 people (40 were women) at the Touch Research Institute in Miami, those who received a 15-minute chair massage at work twice a week for 5 weeks showed lower levels of salivary cortisol than those who simply sat in the massage chairs.

But you don't have to depend on someone else for a massage. We all have trigger points, says Dr. Hernandez-Reif of the Touch Research Institute. Those painful little knots in your neck, for instance. Simply put your thumb on the knot, squeeze, and release several times. "The muscle tends to melt," she says.

Stuck in traffic? Try an eyebrow massage. Pinch each eyebrow, beginning on the inside near the bridge of your nose and moving outward. With each pinch, hold and press for 10 seconds, then release. Or knead your neck, shoulders, or scalp, almost as you would a batch of dough.

Still, there's nothing better than handing a bottle of aromatic oil to your partner and stretching out for a full-body massage. He can use his flattened palms to glide outward along your lower back, away from your spine, being careful not to press on the spine. Or he might rub your feet with the oil, gently pulling your toes and gliding his palms all the way up your legs to your knees and hips.

Either way . . . bliss.

Seek Inner Peace

Jeff Levin, Ph.D., an epidemiologist and senior fellow of the National Institute for Healthcare Research in Rockville, Maryland, has examined some 200 studies of religious participation and health over the last 20 years. He says the studies suggest that certain dimensions of spirituality, such as churchgoing and prayer, are associated with lower stress levels and better overall health.

Dr. Benson has found that repetitive prayer—such as saying the rosary—lowers stress hormones as well as the relaxation response does.

The social support we find at church may also help lower stress levels, he says.

Several studies have found that people who are more outgoing and social have lower levels of cortisol than people who are chronically lonely. "Lonely individuals were more anxious, angry, and negative and less positive, optimistic, comfortable, and secure," researchers report. So just making friends—at church or elsewhere—lowers cortisol and stress.

Try a Supplement

Here are some that experts recommend.

Vitamin C. At the University of Alabama, P. Samuel Campbell, Ph.D., found that feeding 200 milligrams of vitamin C twice a day over 3 weeks to stressed rats reduced their cortisol levels. In human terms, however, we'd need several grams—more than the safe upper limit of 2,000 milligrams—which might cause diarrhea in some people. To help maintain levels of vitamin C throughout the day, take half of the recommended dose in the morning and half at night.

Vitamin B$_6$. This vitamin, also known as pyridoxine, raised levels of the mood-lifting neurotransmitter serotonin in a study of rats at Pantox Laboratories in San Diego. The researchers suggest that B$_6$ may improve mood in people as well. The Daily Value for B$_6$ is 2 milligrams.

Kava kava. In one study of 172 people with anxiety, researchers in Germany found that this herb worked as well as two prescription drugs (bromazepam and oxazepam) at relieving the ef-

fects of stress. Another study found kava kava provided similar benefits with fewer side effects than the prescription drugs.

Herbalist Susun Weed, author of *Healing Wise*, says a safe and effective dose is up to 120 milligrams of kava kava daily for up to 3 months. Weed says kava kava is most effective when stirred and brewed in hot water.

St. John's wort. Another stress-related herb is *Hypericum perforatum*, or St. John's wort. Some researchers believe St. John's wort may stabilize our cortisol levels and raise supplies of the mood-enhancing brain chemical dopamine.

James A. Duke, Ph.D., author of *Dr. Duke's Essential Herbs*, suggests a dose of 900 milligrams of standardized capsules containing 0.3 percent hypericum three times a day.

Stinging nettle. Herbalist Weed says an infusion of this herb strengthens your adrenal glands, thus easing and relieving the effects of stress. Positive anecdotal feedback from thousands of women has convinced Weed of stinging nettle's adrenal strengthening powers.

"When we're stressed, the adrenals work hard and get tired," says Weed, who's also the author of four highly popular herbal books. She buys the dried plant, available in health food stores, and places 1 ounce in a 1-quart canning jar. She fills the jar to the top with boiling water, puts a lid on it, and lets it stand for 4 hours or overnight. Then she strains out the plant material, reserving the liquid. You may drink up to 4 cups of this infusion each day, whether cold, hot, or at room temperature.

Motherwort. Weed says motherwort is much more effective than stinging nettle and calls it "the world's best calmative." She says it rapidly relieves the effects of stress, usually within 1 minute. Weed suggests taking 10 to 30 drops of motherwort tincture in water.

Strong Bones: The Hormonal Connection

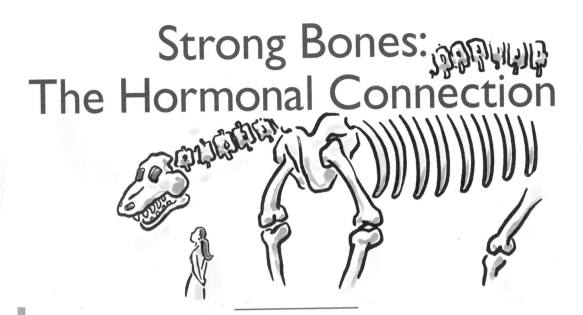

If you've ever pitied "big-boned" women, save your sympathy. Their strength may protect them from one of the most devastating age- and hormone-related processes women experience: osteoporosis. It's a condition where the hormone-controlled process of bone breakdown speeds up even as the bone-rebuilding process slows down. After age 50, half of all American women experience bones weak enough to fracture.

Four to 6 million postmenopausal women in the United States already have the disease, and another 13 to 17 million have low bone mass, just one step away from osteoporosis. By age 90, one-third of all women will suffer a hip fracture. And 16 to 36 percent of elderly people die within a year of a fracture.

Too often, osteoporosis is dismissed as a normal part of aging, but it's completely preventable.

"Osteoporosis should never happen," says Nancy DiMarco, R.D., Ph.D., professor in the department of nutrition and food sciences at Texas Woman's University in Denton.

Here's how to avoid it or, if you already have it, to slow its progress.

Hormones and Hefty Bones

If you think your bones are as inert as a plastic skeleton at a Halloween party, you might be surprised to learn bone is living, growing tissue that's constantly changing. Throughout our lives, our bones break down and rebuild in a process that involves hormones.

Vitamin D (which is actually a hormone our bodies produce with the aid of sunlight) enables our bones to absorb calcium. Without vitamin D, we'd just lose our calcium every time we urinate. Then the parathyroid hormone stimulates cells called osteoclasts to dig holes into the bone, where 99 percent of the body's calcium resides. The osteoclasts release a small amount of calcium from the bones into the blood, where it helps with functions like muscle contraction and blood clotting.

That's when cells called osteoblasts step in, refilling the holes with calcium crystals, collagen, and phosphorus.

Estrogen maintains vitamin D and keeps osteoclasts in line, ensuring there's not too much bone breakdown. Each year, 10 to 30 percent of your skeleton goes through this bone breakdown

CORTISONE AND OSTEOPOROSIS

Cortisone is a hormone that falls in the group called glucocorticoids, otherwise known as steroids. They are produced in the adrenal gland and regulate blood sugar levels, help retain salt and water, suppress allergic reactions, and have a role in metabolism, growth, and the immune system.

But when glucocorticoids are given as a drug, the result is substantial bone loss and devastating osteoporosis, says Robert Marcus, M.D., an endocrinologist at Stanford University.

In the late 1940s, scientists created synthetic glucocorticoids to treat diseases of the central nervous system, asthma, inflammatory bowel disease, and rheumatoid arthritis. But the treatment came with serious consequences. One study found an increased risk of fractures within the first 3 months of taking the drug.

The drug lowers the amount of calcium the body absorbs and increases the amount excreted in the urine. With less calcium in the body, parathyroid hormone breaks down bone to release more calcium into the bloodstream. Glucocorticoids also inhibit new bone formation.

Medications containing glucocorticoids include cortisone, hydrocortisone, prednisone, and prednisolone.

If you're taking glucocorticoids, the American College of Rheumatology suggests frequent bone mineral density measurements during treatment and lifestyle changes such as adding calcium and weight-bearing exercises. Many doctors also prescribe bisphosphonates, an effective treatment of osteoporosis, with steroids such as cortisone, Dr. Marcus says.

"It's as if you're climbing a mountain, and at a certain age, you start going down the other side," says Jane Lukacs, R.N., Ph.D., research fellow at the University of Michigan School of Nursing in Ann Arbor.

The more bone we build by the time we're in our twenties, the better prepared we are for bone loss that occurs with aging and menopause.

So far, estrogen seems to be the most important hormone for bone health, but it's also the most studied, Dr. Lukacs says. "Little research has been done on other sex steroids, so we don't know if 20 more years of research will uncover more information on other hormones and their combined role in bone health," she says.

The Silent Disease

Osteoporosis is called the "silent disease" for a very good reason: 93 percent of the women who have it don't even know it. Unlike arthritis, which is accompanied by swelling and joint pain, osteoporosis has no symptoms until the latter stages of the disease, when there's pain, disfigurement, and debilitation.

Unless you've had your bone density tested, the first sign of osteoporosis is usually a fracture of the vertebra, hip, or forearm from something as minor as bending over, lifting, jumping, or falling. Just opening a car door can result in broken bones once the disease progresses. Bone density is measured with dual-energy x-ray absorptiometry, otherwise known as DEXA. A reading between -1 and -2.5 standard deviations below normal indicates low bone mass. Any reading $+1$ or $+2$

and rebuilding process. It stimulates growth, repairs minor damage from everyday stress, and ensures proper functioning.

But the process changes as we age. When we're young, osteoblasts add more bone than osteoclasts take away, making bones bigger, heavier, and denser. But when we're in our thirties, we reach our peak bone mass. Then we start to break down bone faster than we rebuild it. Bone loss is inevitable.

above the standard deviation is great news, showing you have good bone density, says Dr. Lukacs.

While DEXA is the gold standard when it comes to reliable bone density, it's expensive and usually used only in women who are 65 and older, says Dr. Lukacs.

Other measures of bone density can be used, such as single-energy x-ray absorptiometry, ultrasound, and computed axial tomography (CAT) scans, but these tests involve more radiation exposure, so they're not used very often. For now, DEXA scan measurements provide the only numbers that doctors use to diagnose osteoporosis.

Talk to your doctor about a DEXA scan if you're under 65 and you've had a fracture from a nontraumatic event like falling, if a close family member has had fractures, or if you have another risk for osteoporosis.

If you've been diagnosed with osteoporosis, you should have your bone density checked every 2 years to make sure your treatment is working. Have it checked every year if your initial score was very low—more than −2.5 standard deviations below that of a healthy young woman. If you're taking steroids, get tested every 6 months until your bone density levels stabilize.

What We Can't Change

Regardless of how high our bone mass reaches in our twenties, there are certain risk factors for osteoporosis we just can't avoid. These are the main ones.

Gender. Up to 38 million Americans have osteoporosis, and 80 percent of them are women.

WOMEN ASK WHY

Why do women shrink as they age?

We all—women and men alike—lose ½ to 1 inch of height as we age, whether or not we have osteoporosis. It happens when the collagen disks between the vertebrae collapse as a result of normal aging.

But when height loss reaches 2 or 3 inches, it's probably from spinal compression fractures due to osteoporosis. That's when the bones of the vertebrae become brittle and crumble between the collagen disks that hold them in place. The front of the bone usually compresses first and causes an imbalance in bone support, so most women hunch forward with a rounded back, otherwise known as a dowager's hump.

The compression could be so great that it pushes down on the diaphragm, making it hard to take a deep breath.

Compression varies from woman to woman, but it usually happens in your seventies and eighties. If you have severe osteoporosis, you could experience compression as early as your sixties.

Expert consulted
Carol Wheeler, M.D.
Reproductive endocrinologist
Women and Infants Hospital of Rhode Island
Providence

While one in two women will have a fracture because of the disease, only one in eight men will, because their bones are 30 to 50 percent bigger and denser than ours.

On average, we lose one-third of our bone in the first 5 years after menopause, when our ovaries stop producing estrogen. Although we still get estrogen from body fat, skin, and muscle after menopause, it's not enough to significantly protect against bone loss.

Weight. Here's one time when a few extra pounds can be a good thing. If you weigh less than 127 pounds, your risk of osteoporosis increases. When you weigh more, there is both an increased mechanical strain on your bones, which makes them stronger, and an increase in several hormones that have a positive influence on bone mass. The more physical mass you have, the more you can afford to lose without getting osteoporosis, Dr. Lukacs says.

But it's important to look at why a woman weighs less than 127 pounds. If she's thin because of poor diet, she's probably not getting enough calcium and other nutrients for strong bones. However, there are small, healthy women whose bone density is less simply because they *are* small. These women should be concerned if they start losing bone at a rapid rate, for example, around the time of menopause, says Dr. Lukacs.

Age. The intestine becomes less sensitive to vitamin D over the years, so we don't absorb as much calcium as we get older. Also, bone-building osteoblasts lose function with age, which contributes to bone loss.

Once we lose bone, there's no way to gain it back without the use of drugs. And the older we get, the more we lose, so the more likely we are to get osteoporosis.

Ethnicity. Anyone can get osteoporosis, but Caucasian and Asian women seem to have the highest risk. African-American and Latina women have a lower but still significant risk, with African-American women experiencing one-third the fracture rate of white women.

Genetics. Studies of twins and family members show a genetic link with bone density. One study even suggested that genes may affect the way the body uses vitamin D, thus increasing the risk of osteoporosis. Another study suggests a genetic mutation might affect the production of the collagen that forms bones.

If there's a history of bone fractures in your family or if you suspect your parents or a sibling had low bone mass, you should consider yourself at risk for osteoporosis. If your mother or sister

fractured a bone simply from a fall from standing height but never had her bone density measured, it's safe to conclude that she likely had inadequate bone mass to prevent the fracture. Request a bone mineral density test from your doctor and practice prevention, says Dr. Lukacs.

What We Can Change

Bone loss may be inevitable, but osteoporosis isn't. "There are ways to slow bone loss," says Dr. Lukacs.

Most women know that calcium and weight-bearing exercise lower their risk of osteoporosis, but there's much more you can do to protect your bones.

"I'm always surprised when women who say they exercise and take calcium think that's all they have to do," Dr. Lukacs says.

Don't stop there; find out all the ways to slow bone loss.

Count your calcium. Our bodies need to maintain about 2.2 pounds of calcium to keep bones healthy. Calcium enters the collagen of new bone and extracts water to keep it hard. According to Dr. DiMarco, 99 percent of the calcium we consume resides in our bones and teeth, while the other 1 percent circulates to help with blood clotting and muscle contraction.

But women ages 65 and over are able to absorb less than half the calcium a younger woman can.

If you're between 19 and 50, you need at least 1,000 milligrams of calcium a day. That's about 3½ glasses of milk, Dr. DiMarco says. After age 50, aim for 1,200 milligrams, just half a glass more.

Dairy products, especially milk, are the best way to get calcium, Dr. DiMarco says, because they provide the most concentrated and absorbable form of calcium. Even women who are lactose intolerant can usually handle a small amount of milk at a time—½ to 1 cup—without feeling sick, says Dr. DiMarco.

If you don't like milk, there are plenty of other ways to get calcium, especially with calcium-fortified foods such as juice, cereal, and English muffins. Check food labels to see if you're getting extra calcium with your meals.

But don't go overboard, Dr. Di-Marco says. Try not to get more than 2,400 milligrams of calcium a day. Any amount over 2,400 milligrams may not be absorbed.

Try supplements. If you don't think you're getting enough calcium from your diet or if you don't like dairy products, it's a good idea to have a registered and licensed dietitian evaluate your diet. A dietitian can tell if you're not getting enough calcium. If necessary, she'll suggest simple changes to increase your intake.

Calcium citrate malate, calcium citrate, and calcium carbonate are all effective supplements for women of all ages, says Dr. DiMarco. She suggests two 500-milligram calcium supplements twice a day with food.

Get some sun. Vitamin D is essential for calcium absorption. Just 15 minutes of sunlight a day on your hands and face gives you all the vitamin D you need, Dr. Di-Marco says, but it's also added to milk to ensure the calcium gets absorbed.

Move a little. A small study of men and women between the ages of 40 and 70 found that exercising for 60 minutes twice a week significantly increased bone mass after a year.

Bones respond to the weight that's put on them. If you work your bones harder than usual by walking or lifting weights, they get stronger. You can even target specific bones with specific exercises. The spine, hips, and wrists are three common places for fractures in women with osteoporosis, says Margie Bissinger, a physical

ARE YOU GETTING ENOUGH CALCIUM?

To find out, spend a few days writing down what you eat. Then check the calcium content of your food on labels and this guide. For even greater accuracy, have a nutritionist evaluate your diet. To analyze the specific nutrients your diet provides, a dietitian will likely use a computer program that's not available to the general public. If your calcium intake needs to be corrected, the dietitian will suggest minor dietary changes. To find a dietitian near you, go to the American Dietetic Association's Web site, www.eatright.org, or call (800) 366-1655.

Food	Serving Size	Calcium (mgs)
Calcium-fortified milk	8 oz	500
Lactose-reduced low-fat milk	8 oz	500
Low-fat yogurt, plain	8 oz	447
Canned sardines with bones	3 oz	375
Low-fat yogurt with fruit	8 oz	338
Ricotta cheese, part skim	4 oz	337
Skim milk	8 oz	301
Fruit juice with added calcium	8 oz	300
Bok choy, raw	1 cup	250
Cereal with added calcium	¾ cup	250
Cheddar cheese	1 oz	204
Turnip greens, cooked	1 cup	197
Mozzarella cheese, part skim	1 oz	183
Light vanilla ice cream	1 cup	182
Soybeans, cooked	1 cup	175
Tofu	4 oz	150
Broccoli, cooked	1 cup	42

therapist in Parsippany, New Jersey, and author of *Osteoporosis: An Exercise Guide*.

The best exercises include lifting weights, walking, dancing, stair climbing, and hiking. Women with osteoporosis or low bone mass should avoid the following: exercises that require forward bending, such as toe touches and crunches; sports like golf, tennis, and bowling; and high-impact activities such as jumping, running, jogging, and high-impact aerobics. These activities could increase fracture risk.

But if you have low bone mass and are an avid golfer, tennis player, or bowler, you don't have to quit, Bissinger says. Tennis is a good weight-bearing exercise and doesn't have to be avoided, as long as it's performed properly. Golf and bowling should be approached with caution. (If you've never golfed before, it's probably not a good time to start.) Even if you've been doing these sports for a long time, it's important that you check with your doctor before continuing, says Bissinger. In any activity, be careful not to bend from the waist, only from the hips.

Go green. Studies show that certain nutrients in fruits and vegetables—zinc, magnesium, potassium, fiber, and vitamin C—decrease the risk of low bone mass in premenopausal women.

Eat soy. Soy products like tofu, fortified soy milk, tempeh, and soybeans contain plant estrogens called isoflavones. Just 3 ounces of tofu with calcium may supply up to 60 percent of the daily recommended amount of calcium. Another way to get soy's benefits is to mix soy powder in juice or milk.

GREAT WEIGHT-BEARING EXERCISES

Women with osteoporosis have to pay special attention to the spine, hips, and wrists, where fractures are most common. These exercises, recommended by Margie Bissinger, a physical therapist in Parsippany, New Jersey, and author of *Osteoporosis: An Exercise Guide*, work those areas.

Do each exercise up to 10 times for two or three sets, with a 1- to 2-minute rest between sets. Once you can complete 10 repetitions without feeling tired, strap a 1-pound weight to your wrists or ankles. To continue challenging yourself, gradually increase the amount of weight.

For the hip
Stand and hold the back of a chair or counter, with your knees slightly bent, toes facing forward, and lower abdominal muscles contracted. Bring one leg back to a comfortable level (it's not necessary to straighten your leg) without bending forward. You should feel the effect in your buttocks. Hold for 3 seconds and return the leg to the starting position. Repeat with the other leg.

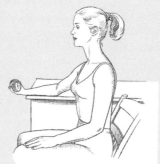

For the wrist
Sit in a chair with your right forearm and elbow resting on a table. Hold a light weight in your hand and allow your wrist to hang over the edge of the table with your palm facing down. Raise your hand as high as is comfortable while keeping your forearm on the table, then return to the starting position. Repeat with your left hand.

For the spine

Stand up straight with your feet shoulder-width apart, your lower abdominal muscles contracted, and your knees slightly bent. Raise your arms as if surrendering. Your elbows should be at 90 degrees and your palms facing forward. Move your arms back while squeezing your shoulder blades together as far as is comfortable. Hold for 3 seconds, then return to the starting position.

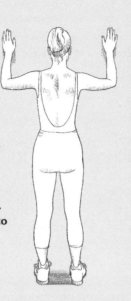

For the back, hip, and wrist

Get on your hands and knees. Keep your neck aligned with your spine while looking at the floor. With your abdominal muscles contracted, slowly raise your right arm out in front of you and hold for 3 seconds before returning to the starting position. Repeat with your left arm. Then slowly raise your left leg straight behind you and hold for 3 seconds before returning to the starting position. Repeat with the other leg.

Once you're comfortable lifting one arm or leg at a time, try lifting your right arm and left leg at the same time, holding for 3 seconds. Alternate sides for the rest of the set.

But the amount of calcium in soy products varies widely, so check the label to be certain how much calcium you're getting.

Some studies suggested that a synthetic form of isoflavone called ipriflavone lowered bone mass. But a study published in 2000 on women with osteoporosis showed the supplement (which was created for a drug trial and not yet available to the public) didn't affect bone mass or fracture occurrence. One surprising side effect of the ipriflavone was lymphopenia, a decrease in the lymphocytes, or white blood cells. White blood cells are a vital part of the body's immune system.

Ditch diets. If you've ever put yourself on a crash diet, chances are you lost more than fat—you lost bone, too. That's because such diets usually cut out dairy foods, the best source of calcium, says Carol Wheeler, M.D., reproductive endocrinologist at Women and Infants Hospital of Rhode Island in Providence. Also, women with anorexia or bulimia who stop menstruating because of dropping estrogen levels often have accelerated bone loss.

Drink tea. Women, especially after menopause, who drink 2 or more cups of coffee a day have reduced bone density because coffee increases calcium loss in urine.

Tea, on the other hand, has isoflavonoids that help our bones. A study of postmenopausal women in Britain found that drinking at least one cup of tea a day increased the drinkers' bone density about 5 percent compared with women who didn't drink tea. Those who added milk had an even higher bone density.

Researchers think the isoflavonoids' ability to mimic estrogen helps maintain bone density in women after they go through menopause.

Stop smoking. Get rid of your smokers' cough and lower your risk of osteoporosis at the same time. Women who smoke may have lower estrogen levels than women who don't, and they go through menopause up to 2 years earlier.

Drink moderately. Having seven or more alcoholic drinks a week increases your risk of falls and hip fractures. Alcohol also lowers your body's ability to build bone. Further, many women who drink too much alcohol have poor nutrition habits, says Robert Marcus, M.D., an endocrinologist at Stanford University.

Fall-proof your house. A low bone-mass screening means a short fall could lead to a fracture, so take precautions around your home and in daily activities. Wear shoes that are appropriate for the surface you are walking on. Remove slippery throw rugs and watch where you walk, especially if the surfaces, such as streets and sidewalks, are uneven. Keep electrical cords tucked out of the way.

Traditional Treatments

Supplemental hormones and other drugs can also help slow bone loss.

Hormone replacement therapy (HRT). The estrogen in HRT can cut your risk for osteoporosis in half by increasing bone density and reducing fractures.

One study found that women who took estrogen replacement therapy alone, without progesterone, cut their risk of hip fractures 4 percent every year they took it. Women on hormone replacement therapy (with progesterone) reduced their risk 11 percent every year they took it. But once you stop taking HRT, studies show, you lose its protection. After 5 years without it, any reductions in fracture risk are lost.

SERMs. Selective estrogen receptor modulators (SERMs) act like estrogen by slowing bone breakdown. This class of drugs includes tamoxifen (Nolvadex), raloxifene (Evista), tibolone (Livial), and droloxifene. The key word in the acronym SERM is "selective," says Dr. Marcus. Different SERMs act like estrogen in some tissues but not in others. Raloxifene, for example, acts like estrogen in the liver and bone but not in the uterus. Thus, it doesn't increase your risk for uterine cancer as estrogen replacement therapy can.

Bisphosphonates. The primary drugs that fight osteoporosis, bisphosphonates shut down the action of the osteoclasts that break down bone, Dr. Marcus says. Drugs in this class include alendronate (Fosamax) and risedronate (Actonel).

Parathyroid hormone. This is a new treatment that was expected to receive FDA approval in 2001. An injection of synthetic parathyroid hormone provides striking improvement in bone density and reduces fractures in older women with osteoporosis.

"It seems to actually stimulate bone formation when combined with estrogen or bisphosphonates," says Lila A. Wallis, M.D., M.A.C.P., clinical professor of medicine at Weill Medical College of Cornell University in New York City.

Calcitonin. The hormone calcitonin has a small role in the fight against osteoporosis, Dr. Marcus says. "It may result in a modest degree of protection against vertebral fractures, but we have no evidence that it protects against fractures anywhere else." But women who desperately need bone protection and can't take estrogen or the other drugs because of side effects can benefit from taking supplemental calcitonin, he says.

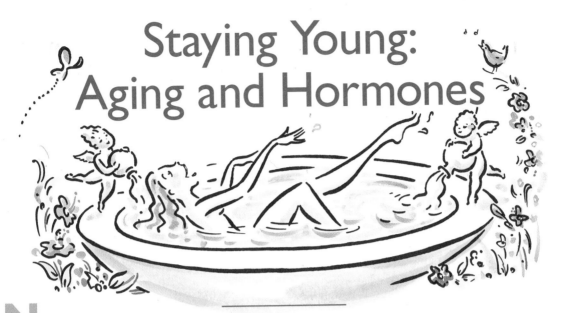

Staying Young: Aging and Hormones

Nearly five centuries after the famed Spanish explorer Juan Ponce de León stumbled upon the coast of Florida instead of the Fountain of Youth he'd set out to find, researchers around the world—including dozens funded by the National Institute on Aging (NIA) in Bethesda, Maryland—are still searching for the fabled fountain. But these days, they're looking deep within us, to our hormones, instead of to the world at large.

Over the past 50 years, they've identified several potential youth-enhancing hormones, including DHEA, melatonin, human growth hormone, pregnenolone, estrogen, and testosterone. These hormones are considered age related because as we get older, their levels in our blood drop like anvils. For instance, from childhood onward, we churn out ample growth hormone until we hit about age 30.

"We're programmed to be that way," says Mary Elizabeth Mason, M.D., an endocrinologist and assistant professor of internal medicine at Eastern Virginia Medical School in Norfolk. "We don't know why."

And so, goes the thinking, if only we could restore those hormones to the amounts we had at 20 or 25, we might be able to restore our youth or, at least, ensure a healthier, independent future.

Recent research suggests it's not as far-fetched a fantasy as it sounds. But that doesn't mean your family practitioner is going to start writing prescriptions for human growth hormone. Besides, you probably don't need it. For research also shows that we may be able to push our bodies' youth-enhancing buttons with vitamins, herbs, foods, exercise, sleep—even friendship.

Living Longer, Living Better

By 2050, thanks to the wonders of modern medicine, more than 2 million Americans—mostly women—will become centenarians. But one national survey found evidence that it's our physical and mental well-being that we worry about as we age, not the number of birthdays we log.

Osteoporosis, decreased muscle mass, plummeting energy, depression, wrinkles, heart disease, cancer, forgetfulness, and Alzheimer's disease are among the unattractive possibilities we face as we check off the years.

Successful aging, then, involves avoiding disease and disability, thriving physically and mentally, and taking part in meaningful social and emotional activities, note researchers John W. Rowe, M.D., and Robert L. Kahn, Ph.D., authors of *Successful Aging*, in an extensive study of longevity.

No wonder that as the baby boomers, the largest demographic bulge in modern history, approach 60, we're seeing "antiaging" doctors pop up everywhere. They offer over-the-counter DHEA, pregnenolone, and melatonin as well as the prescription human growth hormone, estrogen, progesterone, and testosterone. Some promise their potions can restore everything from immunity and energy to wrinkle-free skin, firm fannies, and heftier muscles.

Best to save your money. The FDA has not approved any prescription medicines or over-the-counter supplements for slowing the aging process.

Still, it's worth exploring the research.

The Sex Hormones

"We're still being surprised by estrogen," says Frank Bellino, Ph.D., endocrinology program administrator for the NIA. Perhaps most exciting is that estrogen may bolster memory—or deter Alzheimer's disease, which is more prevalent in

---

SIGNS OF hGH DEFICIENCY

The only way to know for sure if you're deficient in hGH (human growth hormone) is with a blood or saliva test. But the following quiz can provide some clues. Depending on your score, you may want to talk to your doctor about having your levels measured.

Today, as compared with 10 years ago:	If yes:
1. Do you often feel tired?	+1
2. Do you feel happy most of the time?	−2
3. Do you often go through mood swings?	+2
4. Do you anger easily?	+2
5. Are you often depressed?	+1
6. Do you often feel anxious or stressed out?	+1
7. Do you feel you work too hard?	+2
8. Do you look forward to retirement (not to pursue an activity but to do less)?	+2
9. Do you keep in touch with friends?	−1
10. Do you maintain an interest in sex?	−1
11. Is your sex life declining?	+2
12. Do you have trouble falling or staying asleep?	+2
13. Do you feel well-rested after sleep?	−1
14. Do you find yourself forgetting things?	+2
15. Do you find it harder to think clearly?	+2
16. Do you use memory aids (such as lists)?	+2
17. Do you have problems concentrating?	+2
18. Are you in poor physical shape?	+2
19. Are you more than 20 percent above your ideal weight?	+2
20. Is it very difficult for you to lose weight?	+1
21. Have you developed a spare tire or love handles?	+1
22. Do your muscles look youthful?	−2
23. Do you feel your overall health is good?	−2
24. Do you often get colds or feel sick?	+2
25. Do you commonly feel aches or pains?	+1
26. Is your blood cholesterol over 200?	+1
27. Is your blood cholesterol over 240?	+2

28. Is your HDL less than 55?   +2
29. Is your blood pressure normal?   −2
30. Has your vision noticeably deteriorated?   +1
31. Do you urinate frequently?   +1
32. Do you have digestive problems?   +1
33. Does the skin on your face, neck, upper arms,
    and abdomen hang?   +2
34. Do you think you look older than your
    peers?   +1
35. Do you have cellulite on your thighs?   +1
36. Do you need haircuts less frequently?   +1
37. Do cuts, bruises, and wounds take long to heal?   +1
38. Is it getting harder to exercise?   +2
39. Do you have less strength for gripping or lifting?   +2
40. Do you have less endurance?   +2
41. Is your breathing more labored when you
    exercise hard?   +3
42. Do you find the longer you live, the better you
    feel about life?   −2
Ages 45 to 54   +1
Ages 55 to 64   +2
Age 65 and above   +3

                                                    Total _____

Scoring

0–14: You are doing well and your complaints are within the normal range of daily living.

15–22: A growth-hormone enhancing program, in consultation with an antiaging specialist, may help forestall some problems of aging.

23–30: Hormonal replacement therapy with hGH may reverse the problems of aging you are encountering. Schedule a doctor's visit and have your insulin growth-like factor-1 levels checked.

31 and above: Chances are your levels of growth hormone are severely deficient. Hormonal replacement therapy including hGH may be of benefit.

women than men.

Observational research shows that women who use estrogen (outside of controlled studies) are half as likely to develop Alzheimer's as are nonestrogen users, says Pauline M. Maki, Ph.D., an investigator in the Laboratory of Personality and Cognition at the NIA, who researches estrogen and memory. But once women have the disease, estrogen is of little help.

Estrogen may bolster memory in women who don't have Alzheimer's but who are experiencing some forgetfulness as they age, says Dr. Maki. She and other researchers found that women taking hormone replacement therapy (HRT) learned and remembered a shopping list better than women not on HRT.

Additionally, one study using positron emission tomography (PET scans) compared the brain activity of 28 women over 2 years. Those who used estrogen showed improved activity in the hippocampus—the part of the brain that registers and stores information—compared with the nonusers. "There might be something to the idea that estrogen improves memory," Dr. Maki says.

That's still not enough information to recommend estrogen just to deter dementia, she says. But large-scale trials now under way may offer more clues. They may also help reveal progesterone's role, if any, in memory. In one study, progesterone enhanced women's ability to picture an object as it rotated in space—something men are generally more adept at.

glands stimulate hGH's release. It then triggers insulin-like growth factor 1 (IGF-1) in the liver, sending our bodies a message to grow.

By the time we're 70, however, about half of us are totally or partially deficient in hGH. Some researchers believe the drop corresponds to losses in muscle and bone and gains in fat, especially in the abdomen (a risk for heart disease). Young people with growth hormone deficiencies develop similar signs of aging.

Injections of synthetic hGH are FDA approved for children with growth deficiencies and for young adults with pituitary problems, such as tumors. Yet many antiaging specialists prescribe it "off-label"—which means for a use other than the FDA-approved ones. While prescribing off-label is an accepted and legal practice, it remains to be seen whether using hGH for antiaging has any benefits.

Growth hormone has been studied for antiaging since 1990 in animals and people, but the findings have been mixed, say Dr. Rowe and Dr. Kahn, whose MacArthur Foundation research became the basis for their book.

Among the findings: Some women using growth hormone showed more muscle—as opposed to fat—in their thighs and increases in lean body mass. Some of the women also experienced drops of 13 percent in low-density lipoprotein (LDL, the artery-clogging cholesterol).

But the hormone didn't budge their belly fat,

Human Growth Hormone

Thank human growth hormone (hGH) for the fact that we're not 2 feet tall. When we're children, processes in our brains and pituitary

the kind connected with an increased risk of heart disease. And many side effects are connected with hGH, including carpal tunnel syndrome, fluid retention, joint pain, diabetes, high blood pressure, and nausea. The drug is also expensive: anywhere from $500 to $1,200 or more a month.

Be especially wary of anything claiming to be growth hormone that is sold over the counter or any pills or sprays purporting to stimulate hGH (secretagogues). Growth hormone cannot be sold without a prescription, and secretagogues have not been proven beneficial.

DHEA: A Questionable "Fountain of Youth"

Walk into any health food store and you'll see bottles of DHEA (dehydroepiandrosterone), which promises to lift your libido and sense of well-being, erase fat, improve your memory, and boost your energy, muscles, and immunity. Some women use it as a less-expensive alternative to hGH, because a 1-month supply can cost less than $30.

But there's a reason the claims sound too good to be true. There is no solid research proving that safe levels of DHEA supplements can reverse the aging process.

The hormone is made in our adrenal glands as a precursor to estrogen and testosterone. At age 70, we have about 20 percent of the DHEA we had at 25, says Alan Gaby, M.D., professor of therapeutic nutrition at Bastyr University in Kenmore, Washington, and author of *The Patient's Book of Natural Healing*. Low levels are linked to heart disease, obesity, diabetes, cancer, osteoporosis, and dementia. One theory is that DHEA protects us against these maladies by increasing levels of insulin-like growth factor.

Dr. Gaby has seen women taking supplements of 10 milligrams a day show improved muscle mass, memory, and mood within 2 to 4 weeks of starting the supplement. But neither Dr. Gaby nor most other doctors recommend we use it—or its precursor, pregnenolone—at all.

That's because most studies of DHEA have been done only in laboratory animals, says Arthur Schwartz, Ph.D., professor of microbiology at the Fels Research Institute at Temple University in Philadelphia. In mice, it lowers the incidence of breast and colon cancer. In rabbits, it's reduced atherosclerosis, or hardening of the arteries. And in some mice, DHEA has "quite dramatically" proven itself as an antidiabetic, reducing blood sugar and insulin resistance, he says.

But to get similar effects, we'd have to take about 2 grams (2,000 milligrams) a day, says Dr. Schwartz. And the side effects—including increased body hair and deeper voices—from such a large dose would be intolerable, he says.

Ironically, high doses may *cause* the same things low levels are thought to protect against: some cancers and heart disease in women.

Melatonin: Miracle or Myth?

Another supplement plentiful in stores, melatonin is often associated with sleep or easing jet lag. The hormone, produced in the tiny pineal gland within our brains, is thought to regulate our internal body clocks, or circadian rhythms.

But melatonin is also gaining attention in the antiaging arena as a potent antioxidant and immunity booster that helps forestall some of the worst scourges of aging, including cancer and heart disease.

Some specialists speculate it stimulates production of growth hormone.

Even its role in regulating circadian rhythms is thought to play a part in aging. Studies in rats show that body clock disruptions are associated with a loss of nerve cells in the brain, a change also seen in women with Alzheimer's.

One study on a pair of identical twins with Alzheimer's disease showed that 6 milligrams of melatonin taken daily for 3 years slowed the disease's progression. Some researchers think melatonin may someday help treat stroke, brain trauma, and progressive neurological diseases such as Parkinson's.

Despite such results, however, the melatonin studies—mostly in animals—have been too limited to apply to humans, says the NIA's Dr. Bellino. "There isn't any evidence to show the supplements are helpful," he says. "We're not even sure they're safe."

Doctors who prescribe supplements generally use 1 milligram or less. Yet over-the-counter capsules and pills often contain 3 milligrams. Side effects may include confusion, drowsiness, and headache. And too much melatonin may constrict blood vessels, a danger for women with high blood pressure or heart problems.

Natural Ways to Slow Aging

Many simple alternatives to supplementing with hormones abound. They include:

Shake a leg. Dr. Rowe and Dr. Kahn say exercise is the most important thing we can do to stave off aging. Studies show exercise reduces the risk of heart disease, diabetes, high blood pressure, cancer, osteoporosis, depression, arthritis, and other diseases of aging. It in-

REAL-LIFE SCENARIO

She Didn't Like What She Saw in the Mirror

Cheryl, 52, awoke one morning to a vision she didn't like—the face staring back in her mirror. She saw laugh lines around her mouth and eyes. And she wasn't laughing. Even her neck looked like the remnants of a roll of crepe paper.

Years of sunbathing, smoking, and her couch potato lifestyle of junk food and delivery pizzas had caught up with her. "Is it time for a face-lift?" she wondered.

Not necessarily. Start at the bottom of the self-care ladder and work your way up, as you need or want to.

Taking care of yourself is the first step. That means regular exercise, which keeps skin young by promoting blood flow; an antioxidant-rich diet filled with fruits and yellow and leafy green vegetables, vital for cell production; regular sunscreen use (minimum SPF 15) to thwart wrinkle-promoting ultraviolet rays; and no smoking, which destroys cells and skin-firming collagen fibers and hastens wrinkling.

Your body will repair itself. Maybe not totally, but it will kick into gear.

But often, we overlook the simplest of options, like water. Tote around a big bottle of water and sip it all day. Water plumps cells and rehydrates skin.

And, yes, cold cucumber slices placed over closed eyes for a few minutes daily will temporarily lessen swelling. So will hemorrhoid preparations applied under the eyes. An eyebrow waxing can provide an uplifted appearance to the eyes. And a complimentary hair color or blouse may flatter your face and neckline.

creases blood flow to the skin, providing a healthier, younger appearance. And regular workouts also boost hGH and other antiaging hormones, says Vincent Giampapa, M.D., founder of Longevity Institute International in Montclair, New Jersey.

We don't need to run marathons or join a gym

A skin care specialist can offer makeup tips that enhance mature skin. Just applying lipstick, for instance, can brighten your whole appearance.

Moisturizers, too, enhance skin, and some contain sunscreen. But over the years, we may lose the initial luster as we continually apply moisturizer over dead cells. It's like wetting a piece of sandpaper and drying it in the sun. It becomes sandpaper again.

That's where some of the newer skin products can help. To protect the skin and build collagen, try alpha-hydroxy lotions, creams, and peels; prescription creams like Retin-A, which contain retinoic acid and slough off that dead top layer; and products with vitamins E and C in the proper formulations.

But ask a medical skin care specialist before choosing over-the-counter products, which are not regulated by the FDA. There's no guarantee regarding the amounts of ingredients in them.

Another step up the ladder: "lunchtime" chemical peels and microdermabrasions that are done in a physician's office and don't require recovery time. Even higher are Botox or collagen injections to soften lines, stronger peels, dermabrasions, laser surgery, and plastic surgery. In general, with each step, recovery time and costs increase.

Expert consulted
Joyce Black, R.N.
Certified plastic surgery nurse and skin care
*   specialist*
The Aesthetic Skin Care Center
Virginia Beach, Virginia

Exercise your brain. Even mental exercise builds us up—in brain power. Studies in rodents support the "use it or lose it" philosophy for maintaining mental sharpness. Try crossword puzzles, reading, playing cards, or board games.

Get your winks. If you skimp on sleep to get more out of your day, you may be shortening your life or reducing its quality. A small study of 11 young men at the University of Chicago showed sleep debt alters hormone production and mimics the signs of aging.

Just say hello. Research shows that social support—having friends and being around people—promotes long-term health. The study by Dr. Rowe and Dr. Kahn found that frequent emotional support was a "strong predictor" of heightened physical and mental ability. Even a "good, old-fashioned talk," the researchers report, keeps us vital.

To test their theory, the researchers divided nursing home residents into three groups. All were asked to complete a jigsaw puzzle. The first group was encouraged and told its members were doing well. The second group got hands-on help. The third group received neither. In later tests, those who'd been encouraged put the puzzles together more quickly on their own, while the others showed no improvement.

Choose Your Foods Wisely

Food, says Dr. Giampapa, "is the cheapest way to improve your hormonal levels." Eating wisely helps your body make hormones like

to benefit, but the more active we are, the better we'll look (think muscle tone) and feel (think peace). Weight training, especially, builds bones and muscles and helps us maintain our balance. Researchers believe declines in those areas are major causes of frailty, falls, and hip fractures in old age.

hGH and IGF-1, and a balanced diet has been shown to prolong life and protect against excess body fat, heart disease, and cancer.

High on longevity specialists' lists are antioxidant-rich, free-radical-fighting foods bursting with vitamins C and E, the mineral selenium, and phytochemicals. Think whole grains and green leafy vegetables like spinach and kale, as well as bell peppers, onions, garlic, and fresh fruits.

At Tufts University in Boston, rats fed extracts of blueberries, strawberries, and spinach improved in rod-walking and water-maze tests, suggesting that antioxidant-rich foods reverse nerve-cell loss and behavioral declines of aging.

Also choose fresh, cold-water fish (salmon, mackerel, trout) and nonmeat proteins such as soy, which supply the building blocks for proteins that make up some antiaging hormones. Eating protein also bolsters immunity and speeds wound healing.

If your cholesterol is 130 or less, you needn't worry too much about eating cholesterol-laden foods, such as meat and eggs, in moderation. Research shows that when cholesterol falls, so does DHEA. Just don't overdo it, says Dr. Gaby.

Still Looking for a Magic Pill?

Vitamins, minerals, and herbs are among the alternatives to hormonal regimens. Here are some worth trying.

Vitamin C. This antioxidant has gained a reputation for fighting cancer by zapping free radicals and strengthening immunity. Taking up to 2,000 milligrams a day is generally considered safe, but take half the dose in the morning and half at night. Good food sources include bell peppers, oranges, strawberries, broccoli, potatoes, and tomatoes.

Vitamin E. This super-antioxidant not only protects against cancer and flagging immunity but also fights heart disease by preventing plaque that damages blood vessels. At the University of Hawaii in Honolulu, a 6-year study following 3,385 men ages 71 to 93 showed supplementing with vitamins C and E also protects against age-related mental decline and dementia. The suggested daily intake of E is 100 to 400 international units. Good food sources include sunflower seeds, almonds, vegetable oils, wheat germ, and fish.

WOMAN TO WOMAN

Human Growth Hormone Worked for Her

Kelly Nelson didn't feel old until she hit age 70. Suddenly, she didn't have her usual stamina when she bicycled or cross-country skied near her home in East Wenatchee, Washington. Then she tried human growth hormone and felt better almost immediately. This is her story.

For most of my 73 years, I was not active. I never exercised. But in my early fifties, I noticed my upper arms were flabby, and I didn't like it. One day, my husband surprised me with a set of dumbbells and a weight bench. I used them, following exercises in workout books. Within a couple of weeks, my muscles were firmer, and I felt more energetic.

When a gym opened in town, I joined. I also began cross-country skiing and distance bicycling. My daughter, Colleen, and I both lifted weights and became competitive bodybuilders. We've won several contests.

But around age 70, I noticed a change. I didn't feel as spry as usual. Uphill cycling got tougher. I lacked stamina in my cross-country skiing.

Then I heard an antiaging doctor speak at a seminar. He said hormones might improve the quality of life as we age. I was especially intrigued by the idea of using growth hormone to restore muscle tone, energy, and overall well-being.

I didn't want one bit of vitality to slip through my fingers. So I found an antiaging specialist, who performed a thorough workup, including a measure of my growth hormone. It was low, even for someone my age.

I decided to try the hormone, which was shipped to my home weekly (on ice to preserve the quality). Much like a diabetic who uses insulin, I self-injected it about four times a week.

The results were nearly immediate. My sense of well-being improved, as did my energy and strength. Even cuts and colds seemed to heal faster. Everything just came together for me.

But at about $500 a month, the regimen was expensive, and it wasn't covered by my insurance. Now I no longer use the hormone, but the benefits have lasted.

I've not experienced any negative side effects. I also eat healthfully—plenty of legumes and fresh vegetables—and get adequate rest.

At 5-foot-3½ inches and 110 pounds, I have the bone density of a 40-year-old, according to my doctor. And I think my skin looks younger, too. I'm as active as ever—easily cycling 22 miles, cross-country skiing, and training with weights four or five times a week.

I think of myself as a pioneer on the antiaging frontier. The quality of life, not just the quantity, excites me.

Selenium. This mineral helps vitamin E safeguard our cells from free-radical attacks. So it protects us from age-related troubles, such as cancer and heart disease. In one 10-year study of 1,312 women and men, those taking selenium supplements had a 37 percent lower cancer rate than those using a placebo. Participants used 200-microgram supplements. While that's a much higher dosage than the recommended Daily Value of 70 micrograms, it's considered safe to take up to 400 micrograms. Check with your doctor before taking selenium in doses above the Daily Value. Good food sources include fish, shellfish, meats, whole grain cereals, milk, and cheese.

Ginkgo biloba. Haven't heard about ginkgo? Maybe you've forgotten. And that may be reason enough to reach for this herb, according to James A. Duke, Ph.D., author of *Dr. Duke's Essential Herbs.* Numerous European studies show ginkgo promotes blood flow to the brain, helping us think more clearly, remember better, and maybe avoid dementia.

Germany's Commission E—a panel akin to an herbal FDA—reports that ginkgo is a free-radical scavenger that's safe and effective for improving memory. Suggested dosage is 120 milligrams, taken at once or split throughout the day. Because there are different potencies of ginkgo, look for one that contains 24 percent ginkgo heterosides, says Dr. Gaby.

Ginseng. Also known as "root of life" or a "dose of immortality," this aromatic herb has been used for thousands of years in Asia. Herbalists say it contains 18 hormone-like saponins, or ginsenosides, that energize us and protect memory. In his book *Grow Young with HGH*, Ronald Klatz, M.D., president of the American Academy of Anti-Aging Medicine, says ginseng—both American and Asian or Korean—also steps up immunity and improves nerve function and wound healing when combined with a multivitamin and mineral supplement.

Ginseng is sold as capsules, tablets, and liquid extracts. Aim for 200 to 400 milligrams a day in capsule or liquid form, Dr. Klatz suggests, and follow label directions. Be careful, though: High doses may cause nervousness or sleeplessness, or they may have an estrogenic effect after menopause, bringing on menstruation, says Dr. Klatz.

Hormones and Hunger

Think of the woman you love to hate: the thin one who chirps about how she can eat whatever she wants without gaining a pound. Then think about yourself. How you put on a pound just *looking* at a butterscotch sundae. How a hamburger and fries attach themselves to your thighs like Krazy Glue. How is it that our virtual twin sister in height, exercise routine, and diet can stay a slim size 6 while we're fighting to fit into a size 12?

Blame it on hormones.

Yes, hormones. These mischievous little chemical messengers can control what kinds of foods we crave and when we crave them. They tell us when we're full and when we're hungry. (Who knows? Maybe they're the reason you devoured that double chocolate cheesecake the other night.) Perhaps most important, they tell us when to store fat and when to burn it. And as we should've expected, some of these hormonal effects are specific to women only.

But even though your hormones play a role in what and how much you eat, there's no rule that says they have to control you—or your weight. In this chapter, we'll explain which hunger hormones are at work and tell you how to combat them so you don't become their weight-gain victim.

Cravings: They're All in Your Head

Our weight is determined by a balance between how much we eat and how many calories we burn. Despite our tendency to blame our weight on stress, the holidays, or the new ice cream shop, it's largely dependent on the hypothalamus, a part of the brain that oversees metabolism. The hypothalamus does this by controlling a variety of processes that determine the levels of numerous hunger-related peptides, neurotransmitters, and hormones. *All* information relating to appetite—from what and how we eat to how we work off that piece of cheesecake (and either do or don't put on weight)—runs through these processes. And it's a circular system. Even as these chemicals control what and how we eat, what we eat affects their activity.

Galanin: The Fat-Craving Hormone

Take the hormone *galanin*, for instance.

This bad-boy peptide and hormone may be one reason we crave that high-fat ice cream and then have such a hard time working it off. Think of galanin as the fat-craving hormone.

When scientists injected galanin into a rat's hypothalamus, the rat ate more fatty food over the next 24 hours and, naturally, gained more weight. Unfortunately for the rat (and maybe for us), the more galanin it had in its system, the more it stored that extra weight as fat, instead of burning it off.

Further, this higher amount of galanin led not only to a higher amount of body fat but also to overeating. Rats given galanin were never full because the more fat they ate, the more galanin their brains produced—and the more fat they ate. Maybe that explains why one tiny piece of birthday cake is never enough.

But simply eating too many fatty foods isn't the only reason for the rats' (and our) weight gain. Galanin actually causes other hormones, such as insulin and corticosterone, to take those doughnuts we scarfed down and convert them into flab on our tummies and thighs.

Sarah F. Leibowitz, Ph.D., a neurobiologist at Rockefeller University in New York City, theorizes that, even without overeating, the rats gorging on the high-fat diets would continue to gain weight (and fat). That's because they acquired the ability to more "efficiently" convert fat from food into fat in their body—and the galanin in their brains made their muscles burn less fat. Scary thought!

> ### GOT CALCIUM?
>
> A study out of the University of Tennessee in Knoxville suggests that if you don't eat enough calcium, your body thinks you're starving and releases hormones, such as calcitriol, that make your cells store fat instead of releasing it for energy.
>
> In the study, obese mice were given diets of varying calorie and calcium contents. Over 6 weeks, those mice with the low-calorie, high-calcium-from-dairy diet lost a quarter of their body weight and 60 percent of their body fat. The mice getting their calcium from supplements, however, lost only 42 percent of their body fat. Those who had low-calorie, low-calcium diets lost only 8 percent.
>
> Researchers also found that women who ate the recommended daily amount of calcium (1,000 to 1,500 milligrams) lowered their risk of obesity more than 80 percent. But only about a quarter of American women get the recommended amount of calcium.
>
> "Calcium isn't a magic bullet," stresses Michael Zemel, Ph.D., professor of nutrition and medicine and the lead researcher on this project. "But for any given level of calorie intake and physical activity, dietary calcium helps determine what you do with your excess energy—whether you burn it or store it."
>
> Best bet, he says: at least three to four servings of low-fat dairy products a day.

Neuropeptide Y: Craving Carbohydrates

Neuropeptide Y (NPY) is a hormone and peptide that starts us eating, slows how many calories we burn, and increases how much fat we store. But whereas galanin's modus operandi is

Its effects are strongest in the morning, after the night's fast, when blood sugar is low—explaining why a bagel or cereal sounds better for breakfast than chicken pot pie.

It also explains why we often reach for cake and cookies when we're stressed, says Catherine Christie, R.D., Ph.D., a nutrition consultant in Jacksonville, Florida, specializing in stress eating and co-author of *Eat to Stay Young* and *I'd Kill for a Cookie*. The stress hormone cortisol pumps up production of NPY to replenish our stores of carbohydrates, gearing us up for the fight-or-flight response. Exercising and dieting also increase levels of cortisol, adds Dr. Leibowitz.

Combating this type of eating is the focus of Dr. Christie's books—where she notes that "stressed" spelled backward is "desserts." By gaining control over these cravings and learning how to react positively to them, we can sidestep the weight-gain trap set by cravings and stress eating, she says.

Serotonin: Nature's Diet Governor

Aside from making us feel good, the hormone serotonin also has a reputation for reducing appetite. Normally, carbohydrates increase the brain's production of serotonin, and these rising levels of serotonin signal the hypothalamus to stop producing NPY—so we stop craving carbs.

In her book *The Serotonin Solution*, Judith J.

fat, NPY's is carbohydrates, like breads, pastas, and cereals. The more calories we burn, the more NPY we produce and the more carbs we crave, explains Dr. Leibowitz. If we try to diet, NPY sabotages us by increasing and intensifying those cravings.

Wurtman, Ph.D., of the Massachusetts Institute of Technology in Cambridge, suggests it's these carbohydrates that signal the pancreas to release insulin into the bloodstream, which lowers blood levels of all amino acids—except tryptophan, a forerunner to serotonin. Without other amino acids blocking its path, tryptophan has a more direct route to the brain, where it can begin making more serotonin. When carb intake is low, however, so is insulin, and tryptophan has a harder time getting through among all the other amino acids.

The more serotonin we have, the better we feel—and the less we eat. "So many people 'learn' that by eating carbohydrate-rich foods with protein-rich foods for snacks, they can reduce their feelings of depression, anger, and such," says Richard Wurtman, Ph.D., also at MIT, who conducted much of this research with his wife. "You have to eat carbohydrates; otherwise, you're not going to get enough brain serotonin," he says. "When people are put on a low-carbohydrate diet, they get a wicked carbohydrate craving."

He recommends eating a low-fat carbohydrate to boost levels of serotonin. "You have to pick the right carbohydrates because, unfortunately, carbohydrate-rich foods are often paired with fats," he says. "Consequently, this carbohydrate craving can lead to obesity." But, adds Dr. Christie, the effects of these foods on mood (and appetite) are not long lasting—only a couple of hours at best—so expect to go through this cycle time and time again.

Craving the Sweet Stuff

We've been talking a lot about craving fat here, but none of us are actually lusting after a stick of butter or a cup of oil. We're craving sweet and fatty things, like cupcakes and doughnuts. For that, you can blame the connection between the female hormones (including estrogen) and galanin. As estrogen, progesterone, and luteinizing hormone shift throughout our monthly cycles, so do levels of galanin and NPY—and thus their effects on our cravings. Specifically, when levels of these hormones rise, so do galanin levels, sending us reaching for more fatty foods.

When estrogen and progesterone begin to decline, they pull galanin with them—and we crave less of the greasy stuff. But they also pull serotonin levels with them. As a result, our moods change, and we can become depressed, irritable, or lethargic. Our appetites may increase, only now we want carbohydrates.

That may be one reason many women report an increase in food cravings just before they menstruate, when they're in the throes of PMS. Studies have even shown that women with PMS eat and drink more sugary things.

One way to beat these cravings is with regular exercise, Dr. Christie says, since it boosts endorphins, chemicals that provide a sense of calm and well-being. Even a brisk 10-minute walk can help, she notes.

What's Estrogen Got to Do with It?

Just because research shows that women put on about a pound a year between the ages of 30 and 40 doesn't mean we *have* to. Neither does it mean that we have to join the ranks of the 26 percent of women in their thirties who are obese.

As our estrogen levels begin to drop in our mid- to late thirties, our cravings for sugar, starch, fat, and chocolate increase because our bodies are trying to store more fat (a source of

WOMEN ASK WHY

Why did I gain weight while using Depo-Provera?

It's likely that this injectable contraceptive *didn't* cause your weight gain, at least according to the first controlled study that investigated whether Depo-Provera (medroxyprogesterone acetate) actually contributed to premenstrual pound packing.

The study aimed to debunk the myth that women go into a feeding frenzy of chocolate and carbohydrates when they have PMS *and* while they're taking contraceptive hormones.

After 3 months, the study found that while all 20 women ate about 4 percent more food (or roughly 100 calories) during the premenstrual phase of their cycles, they also burned about 4 percent more calories during the same time. And the women taking Depo-Provera actually gained *less* weight during the study than those women not on the contraceptive—who put on more than a pound by the study's end.

Of course, these women didn't know whether they were getting Depo-Provera or a placebo (inactive pill).

What happens when you *choose* to go on a hormone may be a totally different story. Did you start eating more because you *knew* you were on Depo and *thought* it was going to make you gain weight? Did you say, "Oh, I'm on hormones. I must be hungrier"? That's a much different perspective than doing a controlled study.

If Depo-Provera were really the villain and really packed the pounds on, the women taking it would logically have gained more weight than the placebo group. So if you *are* feeling hungrier, it may translate into some specific food choices, but it's not the *hormones* doing that. It's how *you* deal with hunger.

Expert consulted
Christine L. Pelkman, Ph.D.
Postdoctoral Fellow in Nutrition
Pennsylvania State University
University Park

estrogen). Ergo, the perimenopausal weight gain, when some women put on "an average of 5 to 8 pounds in one big whack," says Mary Jane Minkin, M.D., clinical professor of obstetrics and gynecology at Yale University School of Medicine.

"That's the bad news. But the good news is that it's not going to be 5 to 8 pounds every year, so don't go crazy about it," she says.

As we age and our estrogen levels drop, our fat cells may come to the rescue by producing more estrogen of their own—increasing their size, number, and ability to store fat. And if you drastically cut back your calories, these fat cells resist and fight back by growing bigger.

You can exercise until you practically begin stair climbing in your sleep, but it simply won't be enough to reclaim that twenty-something body and combat the inevitable weight gain associated with the "big M." Instead, you need to try to find peace in the fact that this weight gain is essential and beneficial.

"I don't think anybody knows for certain why perimenopausal women gain weight," says Dr. Minkin.

One theory is that women, because of lower estrogen, have less growth hormone, "which is a good livener of metabolism. If you have less of it around, you're going to get fatter," says Dr. Minkin.

Another reason may be our *30 million* fat cells rushing toward The Change before the rest of our body is ready. As we travel through perimenopause from our mid-thirties through our mid-fifties, these fat cells can make our bodies transform "from an hourglass to a beer glass," says Debra Waterhouse, R.D., in her book *Outsmarting the Midlife Fat Cell.*

That's because fat cells seem to glom onto our waistlines. There seems to be a *redistribution* of body tissue going on, says Dr. Minkin. "Most women are making some degree of androgens—the male hormones—long after they make estrogens," which may be contributing to this more masculine shape.

These androgenic substances actually go out to the fat cells, where they become a form of estrogen called estrone. "This is why heavier women are at lower risk for osteoporosis and are at higher risk for cancer of the uterus. They're walking around with their own estrogen factories," says Dr. Minkin. And the bigger these fat cells become, the more estrogen they produce.

But, Dr. Minkin stresses, she's not concerned when she sees a menopausal woman gain a few pounds. "Going from 130 to 180 pounds, however, is not menopause. Something else is going on," she says. If you gained more than a few pounds as you entered menopause, your doctor should take a look at your glucose and thyroid levels to rule out serious medical conditions, she says.

But fear not. As you enter your fifties and move beyond menopause, your fat cells should finish dividing and conquering, Waterhouse notes in her book. Your weight should stabilize, and you might even lose a few pounds.

Feel Fuller with CCK

Ever stopped eating when you hit a comfortably full feeling only to feel like you're going to explode a few minutes later? Again, blame it—at least in part—on hormones.

Cholecystokinin (CCK) is a gut hormone that's triggered when your stomach begins emptying its contents into the small intestine, signaling your brain it's time to put the fork down and push away from the table. But there's a lag time between when you swallow your food and when CCK is released, says Kathleen J. Melanson, R.D., Ph.D., senior scientist at Rippe Lifestyle Institute in Shrewsbury, Massachusetts, and assistant professor at Tufts University School of Medicine in Boston.

CCK teams up with gastric stretch receptors (responsible for how your stomach feels when it's full) as well as gastric emptying (when the contents of your stomach start moving into the upper small intestine). "Foods that make your stomach feel fuller faster may enhance CCK's effects," says Dr. Melanson. So incorporating water, air, or fiber into your meals can increase their volume and make you feel fuller as well.

For example, if you take the exact same ingredients from a chicken casserole and put them into chicken soup, you are likely to feel fuller because the water adds volume. Whipping certain foods or drinks in a blender mixes in air, which may also make you feel fuller.

Eating stimulates CCK release, although different types of food stimulate its release to different extents, says Dr. Melanson. During the time lag before CCK takes action, there are other satiety signals in action, such as an increased blood sugar level (if you've eaten carbohydrates). And since fat empties slowest from your stomach, by the time *that* satiety signal is triggered, you may have already completed your meal—if you eat fast. Then you have delayed-onset satiety and feel stuffed.

Translation: Eat slowly.

No satiety signal works on its own, however, says Dr. Melanson. For example, in addition to CCK, many other hormonal, neuronal, physiological, and metabolic signals interact to tell you when to stop eating, as well as when to *start* eating. Then there are the effects the sight and smell of food, your overall emotional state, and social situations have on appetite. It's a wonder we ever *stop* eating.

But by eating foods with soluble and insoluble fiber (such as raspberries, black bean soup, baked potatoes with skin, peas, and kidney beans) as well as by eating slowly, you can enhance CCK's effect. Eventually, you'll find yourself feeling full on less food . . . always a help with weight loss.

The Insulin Connection

Conducting this band of hormonal effects on your appetite is insulin, which "allows you to use your food properly," according to Karen Chalmers, R.D., director of nutrition services at the Joslin Diabetes Clinic in Boston. If there's any problem with insulin production or insulin sensitivity, it becomes difficult to "turn off" the fat-and-carbohydrate-craving duo of galanin and neuropeptide Y, says Dr. Leibowitz. The result: We eat too much.

In healthy women (without diabetes), eating any carbohydrates causes glucose to enter the bloodstream. That's a signal for your pancreas to release insulin, the hormone that shepherds the glucose, via your blood, either to your muscles—where it's turned into energy—or to your fat cells as temporary storage for later use. As the blood sugar moves out of your bloodstream and into your cells, you get hungry again.

For more information, see Insulin: When Sugar Ain't So Sweet on page 21.

THE OBESITY GENE AND ITS PARTNER IN CRIME: LEPTIN

An ordinary mouse might leave many people squealing and squirming, but an *obese* mouse—weighing three times as much—left researchers excited about the possibility of solving the weight gain puzzle.

Researchers at Howard Hughes Medical Institute at Rockefeller University in New York City found that mice with a defective *ob* gene don't produce leptin, a hormone that normally suppresses appetite while stimulating how many calories we burn. As a result, they had no reason to stop eating and became profoundly fat.

If you give them leptin, says Karen L. Houseknecht, Ph.D., senior research scientist at Pfizer Global Research in Groton, Connecticut, you could cure their obesity.

The discovery of the *ob* gene in 1994 changed the way science thought about obesity. Until then, it had long been considered a psychological condition without a molecular basis of development. Now, says Dr. Houseknecht, scientists realize that "obesity is not simply a matter of willpower or a flaw in character. When anybody—fat, thin, whatever—doesn't eat for 24 hours, leptin falls, and that is a huge, profound signal to eat."

Basically, the more leptin we have, the less hungry we are and the more calories we burn. Unfortunately, the reverse is also true. "When you're losing body fat, your leptin falls, and that's a signal to eat and for metabolism to slow," says Dr. Houseknecht.

So if our bodies are predisposed to *not* lose any weight, what hope is there for the 50.6 million overweight American women? "That's the multimillion-dollar question," says Dr. Houseknecht.

Balancing the Appetite Hormones—Naturally

So what do all these wildly circulating hormones mean for those of us trying to gain a foothold on weight loss? Ah, if only we could

In a later study published in the *Journal of the American Medical Association*, doctors observed obese men and women who injected themselves with varying levels of leptin. Those with the highest amounts of leptin lost the most weight—more than 15 pounds in 6 months—primarily from body fat. Researchers speculate that most obese people are resistant to naturally occurring leptin.

Yet, studies have shown that the leptin levels of people who lost weight and kept it off for a year stayed lower than the levels of those who naturally stayed at that body weight. Thus, these once-heavy people are getting bombarded with messages to eat, even as their metabolisms are inundated with signals to slow. "We might think that if we hit a certain weight level and maintain it, our bodies should 'reset,' but they don't," says Dr. Houseknecht. "And that's the sad thing."

Dr. Houseknecht emphasizes that research into the *ob* gene and leptin is still in its infancy, and leptin shouldn't be seen as the magic bullet for weight loss. But scientists are attempting to fully map how our brains contribute to obesity and eating disorders, which will ultimately lead to novel interventions for these weight disorders.

Other research has discovered hormone-like chemicals in the hypothalamus called *orexins* (after a Greek word meaning "appetite") that stimulate eating. The more orexins given to rats, the more they ate over the following hour—and their food intake tripled within 4 hours. While the effects of these orexins are not as strong as those from the carbohydrate-craving hormone neuropeptide Y, they appear to last longer.

An obesity cure may not be far off. A recent study evaluating 1,320 articles on leptin concluded that it is safe to give to humans. Currently, several clinical trials are under way to determine just how effective leptin will be in treating obesity.

behave like the rats. For when Dr. Leibowitz blocked release of galanin in rats, they ate half as much overall and 65 percent less fat. If this finding could be carried over into humans, we might be able to avoid weight-related disorders such as diabetes and heart disease, she says.

Until a galanin-blocking drug is developed, however, there are things we can do to control our weight and balance our hunger hormones.

Pump up protein. The neurotransmitter/hormone dopamine, which helps us concentrate and focus, may work against galanin. It's like putting a padlock on that basket of brownies, enabling us to eat fewer fatty foods and thus lose weight. One way to produce more dopamine is to eat protein-rich foods like chicken, fish, eggs, low-fat dairy, and beans, suggests Dr. Christie.

Finagle different fats. Sometimes we're not in control of our cravings and simply have to give in, but a hankering for fatty foods needn't be our demise. "In general, we're consuming less fat—a lower percentage of our calories from fat—but we're consuming more calories overall," says Susan Calvert Finn, R.D., Ph.D., director of nutrition services at Ross Products Division of Abbott Laboratories in Columbus, Ohio, and past president of the American Dietetic Association. Reading the labels of fat-free foods shows that their calorie content is usually equal to or higher than that of their full-fat equivalents. "What you want to do is pick good fats," she says, like the monounsaturates found in olive and canola oils, avocados, peanut butter, and most nuts (think almonds, cashews, pecans, and pistachios).

Go for variety. "I think women often overdo it on the carbohydrates," says Dr. Finn. "They need to make sure that their meals contain a mixture of nutrients, because that's going to be more satisfying." Adding protein also helps us feel full longer, she adds, consequently limiting NPY production and carb cravings.

Cut back gradually. Don't skip meals or drastically decrease what you eat, says Dr. Leibowitz, because that could increase your cortisol and NPY—making you want more carbohydrates. Fasting also affects energy levels and moods. If you gradually wean yourself from eating too many carbohydrates and fats, she says, you may be able to slowly taper the amount of these craving-causing chemicals.

Give in—a little. You've got to get *some* carbs in order to shut down that NPY production—it's like the way a dehumidifier stops filling after the water reaches a certain point. So no one is suggesting you cut carbohydrates entirely out of your diet. But skip the simple, often sugar-filled, high-calorie carbs like cakes, cookies, and potato chips in favor of complex carbohydrates like whole wheat breads and pastas, brown rice, oatmeal, corn, potatoes, high-fiber cereals, and even popcorn.

Treat yourself. Dr. Christie speculates that certain foods, like chocolate, may also boost serotonin and endorphins (the "happy hormones," as she calls them). Researchers also found higher levels of norepinephrine—another "focus and concentration" brain chemical (like dopamine)—in the blood of obesity-prone rats, suggesting sugary foods raised its levels. So eating a little bit of something you really want isn't such a bad thing after all, suggests Dr. Finn.

"Treat yourself to something *really good*," she says. "Don't waste your calories on junk stuff. Go buy some really great dark chocolate."

Part Two

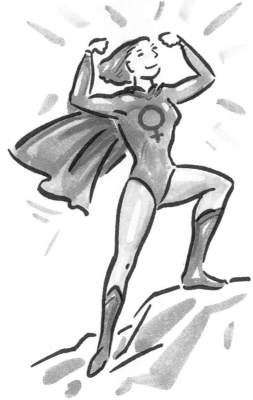

For
Women
Only

Reproductive Health: Take Charge of Your Fertility

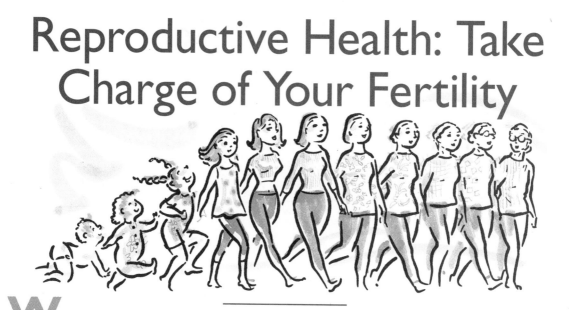

Women are in tune with the earth in a way men can never imagine. Our cycles can be ruled by the moon, the seasons, even the proximity of another person. We have a much more intuitive, cellular understanding of what a month *really* means. We have the capability of stringing 9 months together, sequentially, into a perfect human being—and it is the ebb and flow of hormones that make it all possible.

But sometimes, between PMS and morning sickness, our reproductive hormones throw us a pretty tough curveball, and we wonder: Do we control them, or do they control us? The reality is a combination of both. But there are ways to make your cycles work for you—or at least become a little more manageable.

Menstruation: Keeping the Machinery Well-Oiled

With the responsibility of continuing the species riding on her shoulders, it's no wonder a little girl might feel leery about becoming a woman. Little does she know that her female power actually has its origins years before she gets her first period. By the time she's a 7- to 9-month-old fetus, her ovaries contain around seven million eggs. Of these, however, only 500 will ever make it to ovulation.

About 8 to 11 years after she's born, her estrogen and testosterone levels slowly creep up, budding her breasts, lengthening her body, and filling in the hair between her legs and under her arms. Her brain starts a chain reaction that tickles her ovaries into developing its eggs. After a series of nighttime spikes in follicle-stimulating hormone (FSH) and luteinizing hormone (LH), the little girl becomes a woman.

The average age of puberty in North America is 12¾ years, but it's been declining for the last 150 years at a rate of 2 months per decade. For years, researchers associated the decline with better health and nutrition, but lately they've linked early menarche to everything from environmental estrogens and childhood obesity to relationships with stepfathers.

These controversies only underscore one very clear reality: A woman's cycle can reflect almost everything about her physical and mental health.

PMS: MORE THAN JUST "FEMALE TROUBLE"

PMS is a syndrome so common it's become a verb—as in, "I'm PMSing really badly right now." It's estimated that 8 out of every 10 menstruating women have had PMS.

It boasts more than 100 symptoms, most of which are very familiar: bloating, irritability, headaches, insomnia, weight gain, and acne, among many others. Although doctors don't know what causes it, they do know you have to ovulate to feel it. PMS-like symptoms experienced by women on the Pill are caused by hormone withdrawal, not PMS.

Our worst symptoms often begin when progesterone peaks, about 4 days before we start to bleed. Rather than being a symptom of hormonal balance, PMS is a sensitivity to changes in normal hormone levels, says Ellen Freeman, Ph.D., co-director of the premenstrual syndrome program at the University of Pennsylvania.

Some women's brain chemistries may be more susceptible to the normal fluctuations in estrogen and progesterone. One study found that levels of the progesterone by-product alloprenanolone, which has profound effects on mood, are abnormal in women with debilitating PMS, says Kathleen Light, Ph.D., professor of psychiatry and director of the stress and health research program at the University of North Carolina in Chapel Hill.

But why is one month hell on earth and the next month no problem? Stress and diet are the big culprits, says Dr. Freeman. Any stress we encounter could deplete already dipping stores of endorphins and serotonin, making us more susceptible to pain and irritability. In addition, blood sugar levels can go a bit haywire the week before our periods, and a diet of nutritionally bankrupt junk food or sporadic eating just worsens that condition.

When PMS is emotionally severe and debilitating, it's considered premenstrual dysphoric disorder (PMDD). Seven percent of menstruating women suffer PMDD. Their symptoms sometimes result in divorce, collapsed careers, or even contemplation of suicide.

Thankfully, women with PMDD often respond very well to antidepressants, like Prozac or Zoloft. And fortunately for those of us with standard PMS, there's also plenty we can do ourselves. The most critical weapon in our arsenal is a symptom diary, says Dr. Freeman.

She recommends charting your symptoms for at least 2 months to trace patterns. Then, mix and match a few of the following tips until you find what helps you.

Milk your greens. Winnie Abramson, N.D., a naturopathic doctor in Los Angeles, recommends getting calcium from leafy greens like kale, broccoli, collards, or mustard greens. They also have lots of B vitamins, especially B_6, which is crucial to balancing hormone levels and helping your nervous system deal with stress. Try at least 3 cups of leafy greens a day.

Try a weed. Dandelion is a great all-around PMS remedy, says Dr. Abramson. The leaf is a good diuretic and offers lots of calcium, folate, and magnesium—all good for PMS. Pull up dandelions from your yard (stay away from those exposed to car exhaust or chemical fertilizers) and steep the whole plants for 15 minutes to make a tea. Drink a cup two or three times daily.

Eat right. Eating six small meals of whole grains, veggies, and quality protein, spaced out over the day, can help manage sugar-related mood swings, says Dr. Freeman.

Bliss out with other teas. Sometimes just the act of preparing a cup of tea can put us in the mindset of taking care of ourselves, says Dr. Abramson.

Your Cycle, by the Numbers

The whole menstrual rigmarole was "designed" to make the uterus a spiffy place for an egg to park for 9 months. Your period is, therefore, nature's somewhat messy way of telling you you're not pregnant. For that reason, your cycle officially begins on the first day of your period.

Days 1 through 7. Usually, menstruation lasts about 5 days, give or take a couple. You usually produce about half a cup (130 milliliters) of blood and other discharge, about six completely saturated tampons' worth. Follicle-stimulating hormone, which helps the egg mature and stimulates the ovaries to secrete estrogen and progesterone, rises and kick-starts the 3 to 30 follicles that have been recruited for their big job: releasing the egg. You may feel a sense of relief when your period arrives—the PMS pressure's off, your hormones have leveled, and you're calmer and happier because your body is producing more estrogen.

Days 8 through 14. Here, the whole pregnancy-prepping process is rebooting under your skin. The developing follicles shoot out a bunch of estrogen that rapidly rebuilds the lining you shed last week. Luteinizing hormone and estrogen climb steadily, and a concurrent burst in endorphins helps you feel sharp, efficient, and on top of your game. Your testosterone is also rising, making you very lusty.

Day 15. Ovulation. D day for conception. LH surges for 36 to 48 hours, pulsing many times, and one of these pulses will burst the chosen egg out of its follicle. For every egg

WOMAN TO WOMAN

She Developed Cancer While Pregnant

As a healthy mother of a 3-year-old, Jill Attridge, 35, thought she knew everything about what to expect in her second pregnancy. That is, until she felt a lump in her breast. Faced with risks to both herself and her baby, Jill and her husband, Jack, did the only thing they could—fought for the safety of their unborn child. This is her story.

One night, when I was 30 weeks pregnant with my second daughter, I was watching a show about breast cancer. I thought, "You know, I never check." I did a breast self-exam and immediately felt a lump.

I just happened to have an appointment with my doctor the next morning. He checked it out and said there are sometimes breast changes with pregnancy, but he sent me to the breast clinic anyway. They did a needle biopsy and 5 days later told me it was cancer.

I'd taken fertility drugs with both of my pregnancies, and my first thought was of the drugs. I hadn't had menstrual periods for 6 years before I got pregnant with my first daughter because of low estrogen levels. The doctors thought the estrogen from my pregnancy was causing my tumor to grow—they basically thought I was a walking time bomb.

When I found out, it was a nightmare. We didn't know who to talk to. We tried two doctors in my area, but no one knew what to do with me. They didn't know if they should take out the lymph nodes to see if the cancer had spread or just get the lump out and worry about the lymph nodes later. They didn't even know if they should put me under anesthesia because of the baby.

that's released, another thousand follicles disintegrate.

Days 16 through 21. If a sperm got through and pierced the egg of the month, you can kiss your period goodbye for up to 15 months, which includes breastfeeding time. If not, the ruptured follicle (called the *corpus luteum*) releases progesterone, which reaches its high point 6 to 8 days after ovulation. Although major PMS symptoms concentrate around the last 4

Finally, on the recommendation of a good friend who is a nurse at Boston's Mass General Hospital, my husband called Brigham and Women's Hospital. The doctor said she wasn't taking any new patients for 3 months, but once my husband explained our situation, she saw us the next day. Four days later, in my 31st week of pregnancy, I was in surgery. My surgeon had a senior obstetrician in the operating room, in case I went into labor. She didn't want to wait, and neither did I.

She felt comfortable putting me under anesthesia, and she removed the lump and lymph nodes. The baby was fine, and the report on the lymph nodes came back negative. They wanted to start chemotherapy in case any cancer cells had escaped, so they told me they'd deliver my daughter at 36 weeks. Then they decided to give her another 2 weeks, to be sure her lungs were fully developed. At 38 weeks, they induced, and I had a regular labor.

She was perfect. We named her Kaylin. Ironically, it was a name my husband had on our name list, yet it still enabled us to name her after Dr. Carolyn Kaelin, who'd taken out my lump.

I was so relieved, but it was the biggest scare. I recently had my 1-year checkup, and I'm okay, but the panic is just now going away. When I think about it now, I can't even imagine that I was pregnant and told, "You have cancer." Had I found the lump earlier, my doctors might not have let me carry a pregnancy; had I found it a year later, I might not be doing so well right now. I think I found it at just the right time. We look at our little daughter as a blessing. That's what we think about all the time.

painful at this time. The earlier rise in estrogen caused an increase in the number of mammary ducts, which happens every month unless you're pregnant or breastfeeding. Some studies suggest women who avoid this repeated monthly increase in estrogen, such as breastfeeding moms, have a lower incidence of breast cancer.

The corpus luteum, sensing it doesn't have a baby to support, falls apart and stops producing progesterone. In turn, the uterine lining breaks down, releasing hormones called prostaglandins. These prostaglandins make the uterus contract and expel the lining, causing cramps. Oh joy! It's Day 1 again! Your period has arrived!

Coping Strategies for Your Period

If you've made it past PMS, you just have to survive your period. Here are a couple of strategies to get you through this uniquely female time.

Fight cramps with evening primrose. Prostaglandins, the hormones responsible for labor contractions, are also to blame for menstrual cramps. There are good prostaglandins that have anti-inflammatory action and bad ones with inflammatory properties (which cause the cramps). Winnie Abramson, N.D., a naturopathic doctor in Los Angeles, recommends evening primrose oil (an omega-6 fatty acid containing gamma-linoleic acid), which helps combat bad prostaglandin activity by raising the levels of good ones, diminishing cramps and breast pain. Start with 1,000 milligrams daily a few days before your period begins to head off prostaglandin activity. If necessary, you can work up to 3,000 milligrams.

days of the cycle, you may start to feel their tinglings now.

Days 22 through 28. If there were one week you might wish to opt out of, this would be it. Your estrogen level crashes, taking all of its mood-enhancing benefits with it. This rapid change—rather than the hormone levels themselves—actually causes your body to go through estrogen withdrawal.

Your breasts can be especially tender and

THE TOP 10 QUESTIONS WOMEN ASK ABOUT THEIR PERIODS

1. Why do I crave chocolate just before I menstruate?

"Chocolate has a high level of magnesium, so your craving could mean your body is crying out for this nutrient that's essential for PMS management," says Winnie Abramson, N.D., a naturopathic doctor in Los Angeles. We also eat chocolate because it gives us comfort, a precious commodity in the PMS time. Instead of bingeing, have one or two pieces of dark chocolate—studies show it can boost your endorphins—and be sure to get at least 400 milligrams of magnesium a day, she says.

2. Why do I get cramps in the middle of my cycle?

Right around ovulation, some women experience *mittelschmerz*, German for "middle pain," says Steven Sondheimer, M.D., professor of obstetrics and gynecology at the University of Pennsylvania Medical Center. This cramping may be caused by the formation of the follicle that houses the egg. That's the reason why women usually feel the pain on one side or the other each month. If you continue to have pain, call your doctor.

3. Why are my periods different from month to month?

No one is really sure why we bleed more or less each month, but some of our other varying symptoms—such as cramps, breast tenderness, and irritability—may be due to reactions in our brains to changes in diet and stress levels, says Ellen Freeman, Ph.D., an ob/gyn and psychiatry research professor at the University of Pennsylvania and co-director of the premenstrual syndrome program.

4. Why do I go to the bathroom more often just before my period?

The pressure and bloating in your pelvic area press on your bladder, making you feel like you have to urinate more, even if you really don't have to. Elevated prostaglandins may cause diarrhea, says Mary Jane Minkin, M.D., clinical professor of obstetrics and gynecology at Yale University School of Medicine. Try adding more fiber to your diet—just 20 baby carrots, eaten mindlessly in front of the TV, can add 5 grams of fiber and keep you away from high-fat snacks.

5. Why do I feel sexier at the beginning of my period?

At the beginning of your cycle, brain chemicals dopamine and norepinephrine, which have been

Run away from pain. Exercise naturally boosts endorphins, peptides that raise the pain threshold, elevating your mood and decreasing your susceptibility to pain, says Ellen Freeman, Ph.D., an ob/gyn and psychiatry research professor at the University of Pennsylvania in Philadelphia and co-director of the premenstrual syndrome program. Even if you're already exercising regularly, add a 20-minute stroll daily the week before your period. Walking stimulates the pelvic region, gets fluids moving through the area, and helps reduce bloating.

Formally relax. "Relaxation therapy—especially massage, acupuncture, deep breathing, and yoga stretching—can all bring relief," says Ellen Kamhi, R.N., Ph.D., author of *Cycles of Life: Herbs and Energy Techniques for Women*.

To stretch out your belly and pelvis, try the modified butterfly stretch, says Aadil Palkhivala, senior Iyengar yoga instructor and director of Yoga Centers in Bellevue, Washington. Fold blankets into a stack about 4 to 6 inches high, as wide as your chest and as long as the length from your waist to your head. Sit facing a wall and place the blankets behind you lengthwise, just touching your buttocks. Bring the bottoms of

associated with increased sexual desire, are on the rise. Also, the hormone that spikes during orgasm, oxytocin, is in action, contracting the uterus.

6. Why do I have more energy when my period's over?

By the end of the first week of your cycle, when your period is over, your estrogen and endorphins are halfway to their mid-cycle peak. They bring with them a higher concentration and pain threshold, more oxygen in your blood, and an enhanced sense of well-being, says Barbara Bartlik, M.D., assistant professor of psychiatry at the Weill Medical College of Cornell University in New York City.

7. Why do I become more irritable the week before my period?

The rapid change in the levels of estrogen and progesterone in your body can make you feel like you're going through withdrawal—like coming down off a drug, says Dr. Freeman. She recommends charting your symptoms for a few months to help you feel more in control of your emotions during this time.

8. Why do I gain weight temporarily every month?

Thank aldosterone, an adrenal hormone, for that bloated belly and extra 5 pounds. Because its primary action is to retain fluid, a premenstrual rise in aldosterone can make you gain weight.

9. Why do I get zits before my period?

Some herbalists believe the higher progesterone levels that peak right before you start to bleed are to blame for premenstrual pimple flare-ups. Herbs that promote hormone balance, like chasteberry and alfalfa, can help clear skin disruptions, says Dr. Abramson. She recommends a tea made with one of these herbs two or three times a day. Add I tablespoon of the loose herb to I cup of boiled water and steep for 15 minutes.

10. Why is it so hard to sleep during the first days of my period?

Lack of estrogen may trigger insomnia, and the intense cramping of the first few days of bleeding can also disrupt a solid night's rest. Using nonsteroidal anti-inflammatory pain relievers (NSAIDs) such as ibuprofen can help block prostaglandins' cramp-producing action, says Dr. Freeman. Follow package instructions carefully; overuse of NSAIDs may cause liver damage.

your feet together and rest your toes against the wall, getting as close to the wall as you can.

Use your arms to help you recline backward until your waist, spine, and head are comfortably supported on the blankets. Shut your eyes and concentrate on your breath, inhaling and exhaling gently. Feel your chest and abdomen expand and release. Also feel your belly and pelvis expand and relax, releasing tightness in the groin and uterine walls. Hold this pose for 5 to 10 minutes.

To release the pose, use your hands to bring your knees together and roll to the right off the blankets. Rest in the fetal position before slowly

pushing yourself up with your hands, letting your head dangle and come up last.

Rely on nature's remedies. Dr. Kamhi suggests traditional women's herbs, like cramp bark (400 milligrams twice daily) and dong quai (500 milligrams twice daily) in liquid extracts or capsule form to minimize menstrual pain. Use for 1 to 3 days if cramping is a problem.

Pregnancy: Hormones on High

Your breasts start to hurt. You're feeling a bit tired. You think you're premenstrual, but

MORNING SICKNESS: WHAT DOES IT MEAN?

The first weeks of a pregnancy are like a crash course in the sacrifices of motherhood: minute-by-minute bathroom breaks, swollen breasts, dragging fatigue, and the perennial favorite, morning sickness (which can actually strike any time of the day).

One old wives' tale says women who suffer from severe morning sickness are more likely to have girls—and this myth may have its basis in reality. A study in the *Lancet* on all Swedish births between 1987 and 1995 showed that mothers of girls were admitted to the hospital for morning sickness 25 percent more often than mothers of boys. Study researchers believe the nausea and vomiting are probably due to the hormone human chorionic gonadotropin, present in higher levels in female fetuses.

The nausea and vomiting of early pregnancy may be a built-in defense mechanism, says Althea O'Shaughnessy, M.D., reproductive endocrinologist at the Princeton Center for Infertility and Reproductive Medicine in Lawrenceville, New Jersey. "In ancient times, morning sickness helped women avoid foods that could cause toxicity," she says. The greatest sources of upset are meat, fish, poultry, and eggs, all of which may have carried parasites and bacteria in the days before refrigeration and proper cooking techniques.

By week 12 of your pregnancy, once your baby's organs have developed and it's less vulnerable to toxins, your morning sickness should taper off, says Dr. O'Shaughnessy. Meanwhile, here are a few ways to keep your head out of the toilet bowl.

Hoard that protein. Eating protein can calm the electrical impulses that tell the stomach when to digest (or regurgitate). Rather than the standard saltines, keep a jar of peanut butter or a package of string cheese on your bedside stand to eat before you even get out of bed, says Elizabeth Shadigian, M.D., clinical assistant professor of obstetrics and gynecology at the University of Michigan in Ann Arbor.

Drink in tiny sips. Staying hydrated is key, says Dr. O'Shaughnessy. Sip at least eight glasses of water a day.

Befriend ginger. Ginger tea, gingersnaps, and ginger ale can all help quell your nausea, says Dr. O'Shaughnessy.

your period doesn't come. Then, after downing a spicy chicken burrito, you watch it come back up again. Well, m'dear, it's time to start knitting some booties—you're pregnant.

The first thing your doctor will do is test for human chorionic gonadotropin (hCG), a hormone present only in pregnant women. Levels of hCG double every other day of pregnancy until the fetus is 10 weeks—this lets the doctor know if the pregnancy is progressing normally, says Althea O'Shaughnessy, M.D., reproductive endocrinologist at the Princeton Center for Infertility and Reproductive Medicine in Lawrenceville, New Jersey.

As your pregnancy progresses, your ovaries secrete progesterone and relaxin, a hormone that helps the uterine muscles loosen and expand to grow with the fetus. These hormones continue to rise until you go into labor, when relaxin even helps soften joints and dilate the cervix for labor. Doctors have no idea exactly what triggers labor, but they do know the hormone oxytocin induces contractions, and prostaglandins enhance them.

Our ability to make and soak up oxytocin rises a hundredfold over the course of the pregnancy, peaking during early labor. One theory suggests oxytocin may be responsible for blocking out the memory of labor, so we won't balk at the idea of having another kid. In any case, oxytocin helps us bond with the baby and provide milk.

Boosting Fertility: Helping Nature Take Her Course

Contrary to lectures received in our teens, our odds of becoming pregnant each month are pretty slim. If we manage to hit that window of opportunity at just the right moment, we still have only a little better than a one-in-three chance. Yet some couples try for months, even years, with no success. Before you begin, here are a few tricks to speed the process along.

Do the math. At ovulation, your body temperature rises about 0.5 degree Farenheit, and your cervical mucus becomes thin and stretchy. One drop of this mucus (*spinnbarkeit*) can stretch 2 or 3 inches between your fingers, says Elizabeth Shadigian, M.D., clinical assistant professor of obstetrics and gynecology at the University of Michigan in Ann Arbor. If you have sex during the early hours of this temperature peak, your chances of getting pregnant are much better than at any other time of the month. Monitoring these changes over 2 or 3 months will help you identify your most fertile time, says Dr. Shadigian.

Buy a kit. A home test for rising LH levels is sometimes all we need to "boost" our fertility, says Dr. Kamhi. One woman endured a frustrating year of attempts before conceiving her first child. When she tried for a second, she invested in an ovulation kit—and got pregnant on the first try. "Turns out my calcula-

WOMAN TO WOMAN

Changing Her Lifestyle Helped Her Become Pregnant

After going without birth control for almost 12 years, Rafaella Marcantonio, 33, had almost given up on the prospect of having a child. Then she began studying naturopathy, and her whole lifestyle changed. Within a month of finishing a long period of detoxification, she became pregnant. This is her story.

Throughout my first marriage, we didn't use any protection other than the rhythm method. During the last 5 years, we didn't even do that. I always suspected our infertility was my problem, and when my husband remarried and got his new wife pregnant, I knew for sure.

My gynecologist discovered my uterus is slanted at an unusual angle. A fibroid also made it difficult for my doctor to get access to my cervix, even during a normal gynecological exam, so she said it would be that much harder for me to get pregnant. I also had fibrocystic breasts and a strong breast cancer risk, so my doctors wanted me to keep getting mammograms and biopsies. I thought there had to be a better way. That's what brought me to a naturopathic doctor.

The first thing she did was change my diet. No sugar, no dairy, no mixing certain carbohydrates—pretty simple stuff. I took the herbs scutellaria and gentian with every meal to help with digestion. Within the first 2 weeks, I no longer had stomachaches. Within the next month, I had no cramps. Within a year, my breasts weren't lumpy anymore.

I met my second husband around this time, and he was also interested in naturopathy. I enrolled at the National College of Naturopathic Medicine in Portland to learn more.

Eventually, after a rocky period of ill health, I reached what my teachers call "optimal health." I felt better than I'd ever felt before. I no longer had cramps, skin problems, or lumpy breasts. And in June, I became pregnant. I hadn't been trying more or doing anything differently—my health had just improved.

Many people told me my pregnancy was going to make me really tired, but it never did. I had my son the week before finals. I never felt fatigued, and I know that had everything to do with the changes I made in my life.

tions were all wrong the first time around," she says.

Don't _be_ chaste—take it. Chasteberry (Vitex) helps balance progesterone levels, which are often low in the second half of the cycle in women experiencing infertility, says Dr. Kamhi. She recommends taking 40 milligrams daily of liquid extracts or capsules for at least 3 months from day 14 of your cycle to the beginning of your menstrual flow to help regulate your cycle. Discontinue use if you think you have conceived.

Consider adoption. "When women visit me for help with fertility, I always ask them if they have considered adoption," says Dr. Kamhi. "Many colleagues and I have noticed that pregnancy often occurs shortly after adoption proceedings have been started."

Dr. Kamhi believes the certainty of "having" a baby takes a lot of the pressure off prospective parents, relieving stress that may suppress fertility. "And even if pregnancy doesn't occur, the end result—parenthood—is achieved," she says.

Restart your periods with black cohosh. If you've gone a while without getting a period, there may be any number of reasons. One of the most prevalent stems from an overabundance of hormones in the body, says Dr. Kamhi. While certainly not a cure for serious medical conditions, black cohosh may help balance your estrogen and enable your body to restart your periods, she says. Take 40 milligrams of black cohosh for 8 weeks. Discontinue use if your period starts. Then use from day 14 to the beginning of the next menses.

But if you've stopped ovulating and menstruating, it's important to check immediately to see

ENDOMETRIOSIS: WHEN MENSTRUATION GOES ASTRAY

The same protective lining that can nurture an unborn child can also cause pain and infertility in women with endometriosis.

Endometriosis starts during normal menstruation. As the lining of the uterus is shed, some of those cells get sloughed off and head for the wrong exit. Instead of going from the cervix into the vagina, they retreat back into the fallopian tubes and out into the belly. That can increase pelvic discomfort and cause longer periods.

They then attach themselves to other organs. Because the cells contain receptors for estrogen, they remain very sensitive to hormonal fluctuations. Every month, these endometrial cells grow. The result: severe cramps, painful sex, and high infertility rates.

About 1 in 10 women experiences endometriosis, and the numbers of women afflicted continue to rise. According to the World Health Organization, endometriosis is the leading cause of infertility worldwide.

But how do we get it, and why are some women more susceptible? "Sadly, we don't know," says Steven Sondheimer, M.D., professor of obstetrics and gynecology at the University of Pennsylvania Medical Center. Researchers do know that women whose mothers or sisters experienced endometriosis have a higher risk of developing the disease and that women with children have a lower risk. Mothers' lowered risk may be due to pregnancy and breastfeeding, which offer fewer opportunities for menstrual flow to be misdirected.

Today's rising rates of endometriosis may be related to better diagnosis, says Dr. Sondheimer. Fifty years ago,

if you're pregnant. "Pregnancy is always our first assumption when periods stop in women of childbearing age," says Steven Sondheimer, M.D., professor of obstetrics and gynecology at the University of Pennsylvania Medical Center. Other conditions that interfere with menstruation and fertility include polycystic ovarian syndrome and conditions resulting from hormonal

women with endometriosis were probably assumed to be suffering from severe menstrual cramps or other "female troubles." Now, sophisticated medical tests can pinpoint the problem.

Because endometriosis is stimulated by estrogen, menopause usually marks the end of many women's suffering. But Dr. Sondheimer says you don't have to wait that long to get relief. Birth control pills or Lupron, a drug that suppresses ovulation, could halt menstruation, minimizing hormonal fluctuations that cause most of the pain. If you notice your cramps and bleeding become more severe with age, mention it to your gynecologist.

Many holistic healers link endometriosis to environmental factors, such as dioxin and chlorine. Some recommend using nonbleached feminine products or avoiding tampons altogether.

Herbalist Ellen Kamhi, R.N., Ph.D., author of *Cycles of Life: Herbs and Energy Techniques for Women*, suggests minimizing your exposure to synthetic estrogens in plastics and nonorganic foods. "They can be strong carcinogens and may initiate cell growth," she says. "They also compete with milder forms of estrogen and play havoc with normal mechanisms of the reproductive cycle."

In addition to adopting an organic diet, Dr. Kamhi recommends hormone-balancing herbs, like 500 milligrams of dong quai twice daily, to minimize estrogen's dominance. Or turn to cramp relievers like 400 milligrams of cramp bark twice daily or 500 milligrams of motherwort twice daily. Use for 1 to 3 days if you are experiencing menstrual pain. (Always speak to your doctor if you are experiencing unusual menstrual pain.)

imbalances. Women with these conditions also experience changes in the levels of estrogen, says Dr. Sondheimer.

Breastfeeding

Even before the umbilical cord is cut, a baby's first instinct is to squirm up Mom's belly and search for the holy grail: The Breast.

This instinct, called "rooting," is a good sign for your baby's continued health. The sooner the baby is introduced to the breast, even while still attached by the umbilical cord, the longer and more successfully she will nurse, speculates Dr. Shadigian.

Your breasts grew larger long before labor, due to higher levels of estrogen, progesterone, and prolactin. Before you give birth, they collect colostrum, a kind of breast milk concentrate. As soon as you deliver the placenta, your estrogen levels plummet, prolactin levels shoot up, and the volume of milk in your breasts increases. Over the next few days, your baby's cry or her suckling triggers the release of oxytocin, causing milk to "let down," or come into the breasts.

Oxytocin also helps you bond with your baby, and research suggests it may even improve your resistance to stress.

Breastfeeding's not just good for moms—it's one of the best things you can do to protect your baby's health. Hormone-like proteins in the milk deliver high-potency immunity boosters to babies, protecting them from disease. "I don't pressure my patients, but I say, 'If you can breastfeed for only 2 days, do it,'" says Dr. Shadigian. "It's that important."

If you're concerned about the quantity of breast milk once you're nursing and are considering supplementing with formula, try fenugreek tea to boost your body's natural production of breast milk, recommends Dr. Abramson. Use 1 teaspoon of the herb per cup of boiled water and steep for 5 minutes.

Birth Control Pills: Make Hormone-Smart Choices

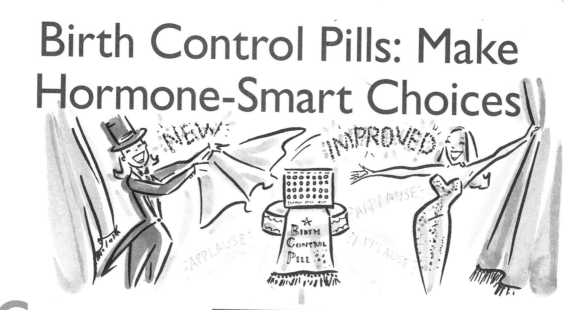

Contraception in prehistoric times: using half an orange as a diaphragm.

Contraception in ancient Egypt: jumping backward seven times immediately after sex.

Contraception in 19th-century America: using a homemade douche made of soapy water, weak vinegar, and various other chemicals that women could obtain and mix for themselves.

Contraception today: swallowing a tiny, safe, effective pill.

For centuries, the ability to prevent pregnancy with anything even approaching the reliability and safety of the birth control pill was a mere fantasy.

But in 1960, two scientists fulfilled that fantasy and changed women's lives forever—spurring the sexual revolution, enabling more women to enter and stay in the workforce, altering relationships between men and women, and for the first time in history, giving women and men a choice about how many children to have and when to have them.

"It was like a godsend," says Susan Scrimshaw, Ph.D., an anthropologist at the University of Illinois School of Public Health in Chicago. "Finally, we had something that was reliable and seemed safe."

Today, the Pill is the most popular birth control method in the world, maybe because it's 99.9 percent effective when properly used. If all the women currently using the Pill instead relied on men using condoms, there would be 687,000 unintended pregnancies a year in this country alone.

But the Pill's value extends far beyond contraception. After more than 30 years of use and research, doctors have learned that the Pill conveys a variety of health benefits on women, from lowering our risk of certain cancers and controlling acne to relieving perimenopausal symptoms like hot flashes. So just because you don't have to worry about pregnancy anymore doesn't mean you should throw away those trusty birth control pills.

Confusing Reports, Surprising Benefits

We might have guessed that the Pill would improve our sex lives, but given years of conflicting information over its safety, who would have imagined it could also improve our health?

"Anytime a drug is introduced, it's studied for safety," says Susan Ballagh, M.D., of the department of obstetrics and gynecology at Eastern Virginia Medical School in Norfolk, a researcher for the Contraceptive Research and Development program funded by the U.S. Agency for International Development. "But because the birth control pill is given to healthy women, it undergoes much more scrutiny."

Among the side-effect myths are that the Pill makes you gain weight. Not true. In one study, researchers followed 128 women who were taking the same type of birth control pill for 4 months. They found the women gained a half-pound during the first half of their cycle but lost it during the second half. The result: The scale either stayed the same or even went *down* for 72 percent of the women.

Some birth control pills with strong male-hormone properties may increase your appetite. But since there are more than 30 types of Pills to choose from, talk to your doctor if you're concerned about weight gain.

The Pill has also been blamed for stroke and breast cancer. And while it's true that the birth control pill increases the chance of a stroke, the risk was much greater with the high-dose estrogen pills of the 1960s and 1970s. Research analyzing all studies on stroke and oral contraceptives since 1960 found that our risk of stroke with today's low-estrogen pills is less than our risk of having a stroke during pregnancy.

Then there were the conflicting reports about the Pill and breast cancer. In 1996, Oxford Uni-

---

THE BIRTH CONTROL PILL: A SOLUTION IN HORMONES

The Pill suppresses your natural hormones and provides its own steady dose of estrogen and progestin. Progestin causes the same effects as the natural hormone progesterone. It works on three fronts to prevent pregnancy:

- Preventing eggs from becoming mature enough to break through the ovarian wall and become fertilized
- Preventing the uterine lining from thickening enough to support a fertilized egg
- Thickening cervical mucus, making it difficult for any sperm to reach an egg

Most pills come in a 28-day pack: 21 pills with hormones and 7 "reminder" pills, which are really blanks. In the 1960s, combination pills had 5 times the estrogen and 10 times the progestin of pills we take today, causing more severe side effects, like nausea and breast tenderness. Additionally, today women who are nursing or who can't take estrogen for other reasons can take progestin-only pills.

---

versity conducted a landmark study to clear up the confusion. Researchers analyzed 54 studies involving more than 150,000 women worldwide. They found that although women had a small increase in breast cancer risk up to 9 years after they stopped taking the Pill, that risk disappeared thereafter. That's true even for women with a family history of breast cancer. Still, the controversy continues.

What's a smart woman to do?

Relax.

"There are just as many studies to show that risk of breast cancer increases slightly with the Pill as there are that show it decreases slightly or that there's no effect," says Donnica L. Moore, M.D., president of Sapphire Women's Health Group in Neshanic Station, New Jersey. "We need to keep in mind that 8 out of 10 women diagnosed with breast cancer will have no risk factors other than being female."

Women with strong family histories of breast cancer—those whose mothers and sisters had it—should consider the newer, low-dose pill (20 micrograms of estrogen), Dr. Moore says.

"There are still a lot of myths about the dangers of birth control pills that are hard to shake," says Marjorie Greenfield, M.D., associate professor of reproductive biology at University Hospitals of Cleveland and director of ob/gyn for DrSpock.com. "But that was because the original pills were much higher doses and had more complications. Doctors also didn't discourage smokers over 35 from taking them. Plus, bad news about the Pill often gets into the news more than benefits do."

And the benefits are plenty.

Top 10 Reasons to Consider the Pill

You may be surprised to learn that none of the following uses has anything to do with preventing pregnancy.

Reason #10: Reduce risk of pelvic inflammatory disease (PID). Usually caused by a sexually transmitted disease like gonorrhea or chlamydia, PID occurs when bacteria in the cervix move into the upper genital tract, causing lower abdominal pain and abnormal vaginal discharge.

The Pill helps reduce risk because it lowers the amount of menstrual blood produced, which acts as a medium for

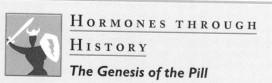

HORMONES THROUGH HISTORY
The Genesis of the Pill

Today, we take accessible, safe birth control like the Pill for granted. But before 1960, negative attitudes toward birth control made it difficult to even exchange information about contraception.

Historically, religions around the world considered birth control immoral. Some branches of Christianity thought couples should have sex for procreation only and that passion distracted men from God. Although Jewish doctrine puts less stringent rules on birth control, it still obligated men and women to have children.

In the late 19th century, this country passed the Comstock Law, which lumped birth control information with pornography, declaring it illegal to publish any such information. The law wasn't overthrown until 1965—after the Pill became legal. So skittish were we about contraception that even the nation's official medical research laboratories—the National Institutes of Health—weren't allowed to research contraception until 1961.

But thanks to two tenacious women—nurse Margaret Sanger, who coined the term "birth control" in 1914, and philanthropist Katherine McCormick—all that changed.

Sanger wrote books, published a magazine, and lectured on the subject. She also opened the first birth control clinic in 1916. That same year, her clinic was shut down, and she was sent to jail for "maintaining a public nuisance." But that didn't stop her from opening other clinics, eventually starting the American Birth Control League, now the Planned Parenthood Federation of America. By the middle of the 1930s, there were 200 birth control clinics in the United States.

But diaphragms, douches, and condoms, the popular forms of birth control before 1960, weren't reliable enough. So Sanger and McCormick joined forces to find something better. In the early 1950s, with $3 million of McCormick's money, they asked scientist Gregory Pincus to start researching a contraceptive pill. Soon he brought in John Rock, a Harvard doctor who was studying infertility in his female patients. Pincus convinced Dr. Rock to give his patients progesterone for 20 days a month.

They discovered that the hormone inhibited ovulation but that after the women stopped taking it, their cycles returned to normal.

During their tests, some estrogen accidentally got into the compound, and the scientists discovered that this combination of hormones eliminated some of the side effects produced by progesterone alone.

They published the first clinical report about the birth control pill in 1956.

Soon after, they began testing their pill on women in Puerto Rico and Haiti. Thousands of women later, in 1960, the FDA approved a significantly lower-dose pill than the one originally tested. Still, it took another 5 years and a Supreme Court ruling before American women won the right to legally use contraceptives.

By 1962, 1.2 million American women were using the Pill. By 1965, 5 million women were on it. Today, more than 10 million women take the Pill.

But Dr. Rock had another struggle to face. He was a devout Catholic but disagreed with the church when the pope proclaimed that practicing contraception was a sin. In 1963, he published a book, *The Time Has Come: A Catholic Doctor's Proposals to End the Battle over Birth Control*. He argued that the Pill was natural because it used a hormone found naturally in women and didn't destroy any organs, but he failed to influence the church.

Still, the work of these four people revolutionized women's attitudes about sex. For the first time *in history*, women could have sex—and enjoy it—without fearing a possible pregnancy.

the bacteria. It also makes the cervical canal smaller and decreases the strength of menstrual cramping, which halts the spread of infection. And by thickening the cervical mucus, it makes it much more difficult for any sperm to carry the bacteria into the upper genital tract.

Reason #9: Prevent benign ovarian cysts. While the high-dose pills that we used to take provided better protection from ovarian cysts—fluid-filled sacs that form on the ovaries—some versions of the Pill that we take today can still help if they're strong enough and if they're used properly. Because the Pill suppresses the follicle-stimulating and luteinizing hormones in the ovaries that cause the cysts, it lowers a woman's chances of developing them.

Reason #8: Treat and prevent endometriosis. In endometriosis, tissue lining the uterus grows outside it, often in the abdomen, rectum, or bladder. That results in severe cramps, infertility, painful sex, and lower back pain. But when the Pill suppresses ovulation, it stops endometrial tissue growth as well. Long-term use often prevents endometriosis from starting. If a woman is already suffering from endometriosis, her symptoms may stop after she starts the Pill. It works best for mild cases, however, with more serious cases often requiring other medication or surgery.

Reason #7: Control acne. You've probably seen the commercials for Ortho Tri-Cyclen, the only brand of birth control pills the FDA has approved to control acne. (There are

WHEN *NOT* TO TAKE THE PILL

There is one type of Pill you may want to avoid. In April 2000, the FDA revised the label on the "third-generation" birth control pills made with a progestin called *desogestrel*, warning that it increases a woman's risk of blood clots. Ironically, desogestrel was created to lower women's risk of heart disease.

But four studies show that these third-generation pills double the risk compared with second-generation pills. Also, two studies suggest that these pills don't really provide any better protection from heart disease.

You shouldn't take *any* type of birth control pill if:

- You think you're pregnant
- You smoke cigarettes and you're older than 35
- You've had blood clots, strokes, or inflammation of the veins
- You have liver disease
- You have breast cancer
- You have vaginal bleeding unrelated to your period
- You have uncontrolled high blood pressure
- You have uncontrolled diabetes
- You have malignant tumors
- You have cancer of the uterus
- You have jaundice (yellowing of the whites of the eyes or the skin)

Make sure you tell your health care professional about the following conditions before starting the Pill.

- Controlled high blood pressure
- Controlled diabetes
- Any risk factors for cardiovascular disease, such as a family history of high cholesterol
- Migraines or other headaches or epilepsy
- Sexually transmitted disease
- Depression
- Varicose veins
- Tuberculosis
- Gallbladder, heart, or kidney disease
- Plans for elective surgery

other brands that have been shown to prevent acne, so you'll need to discuss which one is best with your physician.) By lowering the body's level of androgens—hormones that stimulate oil production in the skin—Ortho Tri-Cyclen helps to control breakouts. It takes about 2 to 3 months for your skin to show the effects after you start taking it, and some women may need to use an additional acne medication. Some other birth control pills, conversely, can make your acne worse because they *contain* androgenic hormones. So talk to your doctor about it.

Reason #6: Eliminate heavy and irregular periods. Because the progestin in the Pill keeps your uterine lining from thickening as much as it usually would, your periods are lighter when you are taking it. And because it helps control your cycle with predictable levels of hormones, you can nearly set your watch by how regular your periods become. No more messy surprises.

Reason #5: Protect bones. One role estrogen plays is maintaining bone mass. Because estrogen levels drop as we reach our late thirties, the estrogen in the Pill can help maintain the bone we already have.

Reason #4: Prevent vaginal dryness. During perimenopause and after menopause, loss of estrogen can result in vaginal dryness, making sex uncomfortable. The Pill, by adding estrogen back in, helps keep vaginal tissue moist throughout perimenopause.

Reason #3: Stop hot flashes and help insomnia. As estrogen levels drop in the years prior to formal menopause (which is when your periods actually stop), the climate control center in your brain reads this as a drop in body temperature and tries to warm things up to compensate. The additional estrogen in the Pill can help moderate this effect.

Reason #2: Prevent some types of cancer. Ovarian cancer kills more American women than any other gynecological cancer. Yet studies suggest that taking birth control pills for just 1 year can lower your risk. After 6 or more years, that risk is cut 60 percent. One theory is that the Pill prevents eggs from maturing and breaking through the ovarian wall, thus preventing damage to the ovary. It is this damage—and the rapidly dividing cells trying to repair the damage—that can alter a cell's genetic code, leading to cancer. The fewer times the cells divide, the lower your risk of developing cancer may be.

The progestins in birth control pills also reduce the risk of endometrial, or uterine, cancer, the fourth most common cancer in women. Because the uterine lining doesn't thicken as much when you're on the Pill—which means that those cells aren't dividing as often—your risk drops by nearly 40 percent after 2 years. After 4 years on the Pill, the risk drops by 60 percent.

WOMEN ASK WHY

Why do women menstruate?

Centuries ago, women menstruated only about 160 times in a lifetime. They got their first periods later than we do, at about age 16, got pregnant at around age 19, gave birth about six times, and breastfed nearly continuously between pregnancies.

Today, we get our first periods at age 12, have our first children at age 24, have two or three children, and breastfeed for only 3 months per birth—if at all. We end up menstruating 450 times in our lives.

But no one can medically say that using hormones to skip periods is healthier. It's simply a matter of personal preference. Some women like a predictable menstrual period as reassurance that they're not pregnant, while others would love to stop having periods altogether.

The only serious risk in skipping menstruation is the possibility of getting pregnant while taking the Pill. Most women know that they're pregnant when they stop getting their periods, but if there are no periods, you might not know you're pregnant for months. The Pill won't affect the fetus, but waiting could complicate things if you choose to terminate the pregnancy. Plus, you'd miss out on valuable early prenatal care.

Otherwise, avoiding menstruation may be a safe way for many women to get relief from painful menstrual symptoms.

Expert consulted
Marjorie Greenfield, M.D.
Associate professor of reproductive biology
University Hospitals of Cleveland
Director of ob/gyn for DrSpock.com

And that's not all. Studies show that the Pill also reduces the risk of colon cancer by 30 to 40 percent. Researchers suspect the protective effect may be due to a reduction in the concentration of bile acids (which help digest fats) in the colon.

WOMEN ASK WHY

What is emergency contraception?

Forty-eight percent of pregnancies among American women are unintended, and half of those occur because contraception failed. But a broken condom or slipped diaphragm doesn't have to mean a pregnancy.

The morning-after pill, taken within 72 hours of unprotected sex, lowers the risk of pregnancy by at least 75 percent.

The way emergency contraception works depends on when it's taken during the menstrual cycle. It can change the uterine lining to prevent a fertilized egg from implanting. Or it may delay or inhibit ovulation or prevent the transport of the egg and sperm.

Emergency contraception is *not* the same thing as abortion. In fact, the pills won't work if a fertilized egg has already moved from the fallopian tubes and implanted into the uterine lining (typically 5 to 7 days after fertilization).

There are no long-term or serious side effects from emergency contraception, but half of all women who take it feel nauseated and about 20 percent vomit—therefore, your physician may recommend an antinausea prescription. The pills could also cause fatigue, dizziness, headaches, or breast tenderness.

Although emergency contraception has been around for 25 years, many women don't know it exists. According to a 1997 survey, only 11 percent of women had heard about it, knew that it could be used within 72 hours of intercourse, and realized they could get it in the United States.

Any physician who can prescribe the Pill can prescribe emergency contraception, so call your doctor—even if it's on the weekend—as soon as you think you need it. For a list of providers, go to http://ec.princeton.edu and click on the directory of providers under "Where Can I Find Emergency Contraception?" Follow the directions.

Expert consulted
Sharon Winer, M.D.
Clinical professor of obstetrics and gynecology
University of Southern California
Los Angeles

Reason #1: Improve your sex life. Some types of birth control pills may increase your libido because they have progestins, which act like male hormones, says Dr. Moore. Although androgens, such as testosterone, may produce some side effects you don't want (like acne), they can also increase sex drive.

Also, if you have low levels of natural estrogen, your sex drive is probably going to be pretty low as well. So the added estrogen in the birth control pill increases your level of estrogen and helps you feel sexier, says Dr. Moore. Plus, feeling secure about contraception can make you feel more relaxed about sex.

And if you're perimenopausal and your natural hormone levels are on a roller coaster, you'll probably experience hot flashes, night sweats, vaginal dryness, and irritability—all very *un*sexy side effects. When you take birth control pills, however, your estrogen levels balance out, side effects become less severe or go away completely, and you'll probably get a libido boost.

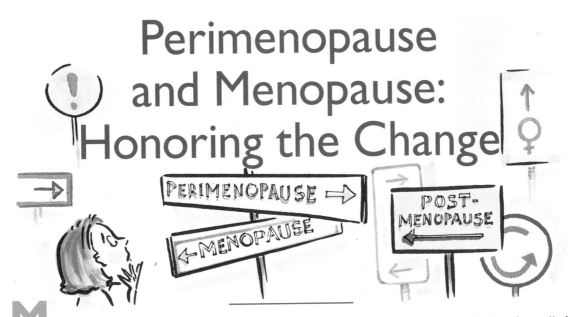

Perimenopause and Menopause: Honoring the Change

Modern women do many things our grand-mothers never dreamed of—ride whitewater rapids, work shoulder to shoulder with men, and postpone or entirely bypass childbearing. However, unlike our foremothers of a century ago, whose average life expectancy was 47, women today can expect to live at least 30 years beyond menopause. And while the very term "post-menopausal" fills many women with anxiety, even dread, we'd probably all agree it sure beats the alternative.

Within the next two decades, a menopausal wave will deposit on society's shore the largest population of postreproductive women history has ever seen. About 40 million American women will reach menopause by the year 2020, according to the North American Menopause Society (NAMS), based in Cleveland. The challenge facing all of us is how to define our postreproductive life.

Menopause: The Day

Menopause is actually only one day in your life—the 365th day from the date of your last period. It's the years that precede that day, called *perimenopause*, that can drive us nuts—or not. For menopause, contrary to popular perception, is not a disease but a natural event affecting every woman differently.

And just as with menstruation, no matter what your friends who go through it first tell you, your experience will be unique. For some, the end of fertility (and the end of concerns about birth control and menstrual periods) brings a sense of freedom. It becomes a bridge to a time of life when many women report feeling more confident, empowered, involved, and energized than in their younger years.

This vital life passage has been long misunderstood, traditionally ignored, and not openly discussed until very recently, says Adelaide Nardone, M.D., a gynecologist in Mount Kisco, New York, and medical advisor for the Vagisil Women's Health Center. Yet most women today will live a third of their lives in the postmenopausal period, she says. Negotiating the hormonal tides this stage of life brings will determine how healthy and vital the rest of your life will be, she says, noting there is no "one size

10 Myths of Menopause

1. Menopause makes you crazy. Perhaps the most pervasive myth associated with menopause is that mental health problems result from decreased hormone production. No scientific research shows that natural menopause is responsible for true clinical depression, anxiety, severe memory lapses, or erratic behavior.

2. Your age when you first started menstruating determines your age when menopause begins. Contrary to folklore, age at onset of menstruation plays no part. Nor does your contraceptive or sexual history.

3. Menopause can be cured. Many doctors have approached menopause as if it were an estrogen deficiency disease. It's not. This is a natural transition, and while hormone replacement therapy (HRT) can ease unpleasant side effects, it can't turn back the hands of time.

4. All the physical changes associated with menopause are bad. Just consider: No more estrogen-stoked migraines. No more PMS. No more debilitating cramps. Lots of women who've suffered these ailments agree "menopause is probably the best thing that ever happened to me." P.S.: No more concerns about pregnancy and birth control either.

5. Menopause makes you irritable. Night sweats and hot flashes may disrupt healthy sleep patterns, as can falling estrogen levels. Without enough deep sleep, anyone can feel tired and cranky, but it's a myth that menopause itself makes you irritable.

6. You're no longer a "real" woman. If you feel this way, retool your self-image and realize you're a person whose value has to do with a great deal more than the ability to make babies, says Patricia Love, Ed.D., a relationship therapist in Austin, Texas. You are more than a uterus. Act like it.

7. Menopause makes you lose interest in sex. Previous attitudes often dictate a woman's view of her sexuality as she ages. In general, women who enjoyed sex in their younger years will continue to do so during midlife and beyond, says Dr. Love, noting that many women in their seventies and eighties enjoy satisfying sex lives. With age, there's a gradual decline in sexual drive for both women and men. However, a decline does not mean an abrupt halt.

8. The best years are over. Ovarian failure doesn't mean your mind, your humanity, and your spirit stop growing. People don't simply fossilize. A majority of menopausal women today believe these are the best years of their lives.

9. Menopause makes you unattractive. Beauty, grace, and allure are not a function of age or fertility. European women are considered attractive well into their sixth and seventh decades, notes Dr. Love. Think of Sophia Loren.

10. Energy drops after menopause. Actually, it's the opposite. Hormone cycling is an enormous energy drain. Women exhibit extraordinary stamina after menopause, says Dr. Love, especially if they exercise and eat right.

fits all approach" because every woman is different.

Your attitude toward aging largely determines the quality of your postmenopausal life, says Dr. Nardone. She encourages women to view menopause as a transition from a healthy reproductive life to a healthy nonreproductive life. If we see ourselves as dynamic individuals rather than simply as child bearers, she says, "this stage of life will be as fulfilling as the reproductive years."

PERIMENOPAUSE AND MENOPAUSE: HONORING THE CHANGE

There are some tricky eddies to negotiate, though. In a society that exalts youthful beauty, women approaching menopause begin to feel invisible as wrinkles appear and bodies thicken. Mass culture bombards us with negative messages about aging, telling us that once we pass a "certain age" we're undesirable and useless, leaving many of us wondering "Who, and what, am I if I'm no longer young?"

Fortunately, as the many baby boomers—those born between 1946 and 1964—move through this change of life, they're altering perceptions and reframing menopause in a positive light. More and more women are shedding the view that menopause marks the end of their lives as "real women" and realizing that the energy not expended on hormonal upheavals can be channeled into a gloriously fulfilling new life.

They're learning to live, as anthropologist Margaret Mead described it, with PMZ: Postmenopausal Zeal.

Menopause: A Time of Transition

Menopause is triggered when your ovaries slow their production of the female sex hormones estrogen and progesterone.

Estrogen, the hormone responsible for making us women, is predominantly produced in the ovaries. It has many receptor sites in the fe-

MALE MENOPAUSE: MYTH OR REALITY?

Reality, says Marc R. Rose, M.D., a specialist in antiaging medicine and author of *A Woman's Guide to Male Menopause*. Male menopause has a more gradual onset than the female version. As a result, when men express concern about flagging energy or sexual dysfunction, doctors usually tell them these changes are an inevitable part of aging.

Fertility may not be dramatically affected, but men begin experiencing significant hormonal declines by their mid-thirties. Androgens, male hormones produced largely by the testicles, start dropping off, affecting sex drive, energy levels, mood, and muscle tone.

Testosterone and DHEA (dehydroepiandrosterone) are the main androgens related to "andropause," the term given to the accelerating hormonal transformation men experience in their forties and fifties. Total testosterone levels, as measured in the bloodstream, decrease at the rate of about 1 percent per year.

While the overall testosterone decline is gradual, the real kicker is the drop in free testosterone. As men age, levels of a protein called sex hormone binding globulin (SHBG) increase. This protein binds with testosterone in the bloodstream and makes it unavailable to tissues. It's the free testosterone—the hormone *not* bound to SHBG—that provides beneficial effects, including cardiovascular protection. Simply put, as a man ages, his body's mechanism for freeing enough testosterone to keep him youthful begins to fail.

Levels of DHEA, the building block for many other hormones, including testosterone, also peak at about age 25 and then start to decline slowly, hitting bottom at 10 to 20 percent of peak concentrations in later life. The lower the DHEA levels, the higher the risk of just about any illness related to aging.

The drastic changes of andropause can be offset by hormone supplements monitored by a physician. Several studies have shown that giving testosterone and DHEA to men with low naturally occurring levels of these hormones significantly improves their mood, energy, and sexual desire.

WOMEN ASK WHY

How can I help my husband through my menopause?

The more a man can ease his wife's menopause journey, the easier it will be on him. Helping your husband through your menopause starts with negotiating for your needs. Yet many of us are not very good at saying clearly and distinctly what we need. We expect our spouses to somehow *know*, leaving them feeling angry and frustrated when their efforts fall short.

Women who are sensitive to their own needs, as well as the needs of their partners, generally feel better about themselves. And most husbands will come through if their wives tell them how to help. Here are some suggestions.

Express your need for his support, then give him specific direction. If you're feeling fat, bloated, and cranky, and sex is the furthest thing from your mind, let him know how you feel and tell him you expect him to honor your condition. The physical and emotional discomfort you're experiencing is real, and you deserve to be treated kindly. When he treats you that way, express appreciation for his caring.

Tell him you need reassurance, but remember that he needs reassurance, too. Even if you're bouncing off the walls emotionally, be sure to let him know it's not personal. Right now, you can't tend to his hurt feelings, so he should QTIP (quit taking it personally).

Take steps to make domestic duties more equitable. Women are used to doing so much and never asking for help. Yet inside, they're resentful, which makes them irritable—which, in turn, makes them more prone to menopausal meltdown. Most men want to be helpful, but they're not sure how.

Tell your husband how he can lighten your household load. Then, when he does these jobs, don't criticize; towels folded in half are fine, even if you always fold them in thirds.

Expert consulted
Patricia Love, Ed.D.
Austin, Texas
Coauthor of Hot Monogamy: Essential Steps
    to More Passionate, Intimate Lovemaking

male body, including the uterus, vagina, breasts, bones, skin, and even the brain. Estrogen levels have highs and lows at different stages of female development, dropping off gradually during perimenopause and declining significantly at menopause.

Progesterone, also produced predominantly in the ovaries, keeps estrogen in check, particularly in the uterus. It acts as an antiestrogen, so the uterine lining doesn't overgrow, a risk factor for uterine cancer.

The average age of natural menopause in this country is 51 (a figure that hasn't changed much over the past few centuries), but some women reach menopause in their thirties and a few in their sixties. Women who smoke tend to reach menopause a year or two earlier than nonsmokers. Overweight women tend to have a later menopause.

Menopause before age 40 is considered premature. There can be several causes, including genetics and autoimmune disorders. If you are experiencing signs of menopause—hot flashes, night sweats, or missed periods—see your doctor for a complete evaluation.

Induced menopause can occur at any age due to surgical removal of the ovaries or damage to the ovaries from treatments like chemotherapy and radiation.

Natural menopause, however, is a gradual process, a journey that takes years to navigate. Most women notice their bodies beginning to change in their mid-thirties. As ovarian function decreases, hormone production becomes erratic and diminishes, causing disruptions in the menstrual cycle and the onset of symptoms such as hot flashes. Most women begin experiencing these symptoms 2 to 10 years before menstrual periods end. These years mark the *perimenopause.*

This is probably the least understood and most misdiagnosed stage of a woman's life, says Dr. Nardone. The hellish change of life many women associate with menopause is actually misunderstood perimenopause, she says. "Since the changes are often subtle and inconsistent, many women cannot pinpoint exactly what they are feeling or what is wrong. They just know they're feeling bad. People need to realize that the feelings women have at this time are not just emotional but the result of actual endocrinologic alterations in their bodies."

As estrogen levels wane, we may find ourselves plagued by an array of stressful symptoms. These include:

Menstrual cycle disruptions. These may include lighter or heavier bleeding, and longer, shorter, or skipped periods.

Hot flashes. The hallmark symptom of plummeting estrogen, they affect 65 percent of perimenopausal women. These personal heat waves start in the center of your body, then a flash of heat spreads like a wall of flame to the top of your head, flushing your face, neck, and arms a fiery red and making

WOMEN ASK WHY

Why did I start snoring only after menopause?

When women suddenly start snoring, it's a definite sign that estrogen is plummeting. As this hormone drops, it affects the sensory nerves in the soft palate, causing it to lose muscle tone and become flaccid. As you sleep, the soft palate flaps, creating the lovely sound known as snoring.

There are other factors at work as well. Menopausal weight gain, also known as "the Buddha belly," crowds the internal organs, pushing them up and putting pressure on the diaphragm. You have to work harder to breathe, and the force of the air in and out causes you to snore.

Hypothyroidism is another culprit. A sluggish thyroid aggravates sinus problems, plus it contributes to weight gain. Menopause triggers hypothyroidism in many women; by age 70, about 70 percent of all American women have an underactive thyroid.

So what can you do, short of buying your spouse earplugs?

- Elevate your head to reduce soft palate flapping.

- Use a low-dose, over-the-counter decongestant at night to keep sinus clogs at bay. Take the smallest dose you can since decongestants can keep some people awake.

- If you're on estrogen replacement therapy, take it at night. This will enhance sleep, taking you to a deeper level faster.

- Have your thyroid tested. If it's low, have your doctor prescribe medication to supplement lacking thyroid hormone.

- Avoid excess soy isoflavones in your diet. Although they're being promoted as a natural replacement for estrogen, they aren't, and eating more than 40 milligrams a day may increase your risk of developing hypothyroidism.

Expert consulted
Larrian Gillespie, M.D.
Los Angeles
Author of The Menopause Diet

your skin warm to the touch. They can last from seconds to 30 minutes and are accompanied by increased heart rate, shallow breathing, and sweating. Chills and exhaustion usually follow. And the fun part: Hot flashes can occur as often as 50 times a day in extreme cases.

Night sweats. These are hot flashes that occur during sleep. You wake drenched in sweat, sometimes several times a night. Because they disturb sleep, you're often tired during the day.

Vaginal atrophy. Estrogen loss causes the tissues of the vagina to become dry, thin, and less elastic. Sex often becomes painful, although over-the-counter vaginal moisturizers and lubricants can help. The vagina can also become inflamed and irritated from a high alkaline content (a vaginal pH above 7), resulting in a condition called atrophic vaginitis. The higher pH can also make you more prone to infection.

Urinary tract changes. You may need to urinate more often because the lining of the urethra is thinning and the surrounding pelvic muscles grow weaker. Incontinence may become a problem, or you may experience frequent bladder infections, painful urination, or the need to "go" several times during the night.

Diminished sex drive. In addition to losing their ability to secrete estrogen, your ovaries no longer produce testosterone, the hormone responsible for sex drive. Some women may continue to produce the tiny amount needed through the adrenal glands.

Forgetfulness. This is one of the most common complaints from women in peri-

WOMEN ASK WHY

Why am I getting more fat around my middle now that I'm 55?

Even medical experts can't agree whether it's aging or menopause that causes extra pounds to migrate toward the middle. They just know that the average American woman puts on up to 15 pounds during late adulthood, most of it around her waist. One reason is that aging causes your metabolism to slow down and your lean muscle mass to decrease. Since lean muscle cells burn more calories than fat, the less muscle you have, the fewer calories you burn. Add to this the fact that the shape of your body is determined by muscle strength and it's no surprise that as muscles grow weaker, paunches start.

Now think back to puberty and childbirth, two other major hormonal shifts in your life. Both events triggered changes in body composition and weight. Menopause is no different, except that as your estrogen decreases, a subsequent increase in insulin makes losing weight more difficult.

Even women who don't gain weight can see 10 to 15 pounds shift to the waist, an effect of aging known as "central obesity." Osteoporosis magnifies the problem, as it causes the spine to shrink, shortening the waistline.

Besides making you feel unattractive, extra pounds around your middle are sometimes associated with cardiovascular disease, hypertension, and an increased breast cancer risk. The best way to combat abdominal spread? Sensible eating and exercise.

menopause. For many, frequent memory lapses, sudden blanks, and forgotten names can be scary and may lead them to believe they're not as sharp as they used to be.

Emotional changes. Irritability, mood swings, anxiety, and depression are frequently the result of fluctuating hormones. But they can also be completely unrelated to hormonal shifts, Dr. Nardone cautions, so discuss any lingering

Don't deprive yourself of too many calories or your body will go into starvation mode, which lowers your metabolism even more. Follow a low-fat diet and do some kind of aerobic exercise for at least 30 minutes three times a week to boost your metabolism and burn fat. Weight-bearing exercise, like walking, will also strengthen your bones and prevent osteoporosis.

And don't look to hormone replacement therapy (HRT) as some kind of magic answer. Research to date is inconclusive. One study found that women on HRT gained more weight than those not on HRT, while another found that HRT appeared to prevent the increase in abdominal fat. Any decision regarding HRT should be based on your overall health, not on your desire to lose weight.

As you move through menopause, try not to curse your fat cells. They help convert other chemicals in your body into estrogen, which may ease your transition by reducing the incidence and severity of hot flashes, mood swings, and sleep disturbances.

And if ever there is a time to accept yourself, menopause is it. Concentrate on being fit and healthy rather than squeezing into your jeans from college.

Expert consulted
Adelaide Nardone, M.D.
Gynecologist
Mount Kisco, New York
Medical advisor for the Vagisil Women's
*   Health Center*

climacteric. About 75 percent of women experience more than one of these symptoms from perimenopause to postmenopause.

Still, decreasing hormone levels don't always translate to misery. Studies show that only 25 to 30 percent of women seek medical attention for menopausal symptoms. The rest either tolerate their discomfort or simply don't experience anything annoying enough to warrant attention. Because symptoms come on gradually and can be very subtle, you may not realize at first that they're all connected to the same thing—declining and fluctuating levels of estrogen and progesterone.

Is It Menopause or Just a Really Bad Day?

The only way to know for sure if you're in the perimenopause transition or if you have reached menopause is with a visit to your doctor. She will rule out pregnancy or serious health problems like uterine cancer and take a blood test to assess your estrogen levels.

The most reliable test measures the level of follicle-stimulating hormone (FSH), a hormone secreted by the pituitary gland to stimulate estrogen production. As the ovaries' estrogen production decreases, the pituitary gland increases production of FSH. Levels of 30 to 40 mIU/mL or above mean you've reached menopause. Levels from 10 to near 30 mean there's still partial ovarian function.

Even FSH levels, however, can sometimes be misleading. They tend to fluctuate month to month during perimenopause. To confirm

emotional changes with your physician or a therapist.

Formication. This is the bizarre sensation that ants are crawling over your skin. It occurs in about 20 percent of women.

Hair loss, insomnia, and general feminine itching. These other common symptoms of estrogen loss can continue for up to 3 years following your last period, a time known as the

BLAME IT ON HORMONES

Fading Memory

You walk into the living room to get something, but what? You drive right past your son's school and forget to turn in. What's going on?

The connection between memory and menopause has long been an issue of debate. Ongoing research into brain function is trying to determine whether estrogen receptors or estrogen metabolites (the breakdown products of estrogen) affect memory function. But so far, nothing has been proven, says gynecologist Adelaide Nardone, M.D., of Mount Kisco, New York.

Recent research at Yale University used magnetic resonance imaging (MRI) to study the influence of estrogen on the brain patterns of postmenopausal women. Therapeutic doses of estrogen affected brain activity in memory tasks, like remembering a just-looked-up telephone number, which seems to support the theory that estrogen aids short-term information storage.

This small study provides a tantalizing clue to estrogen's role in brain function, but definitive links have not been forged, says Dr. Nardone, who believes that much of menopausal "mental misfiring" can be traced to fatigue.

Women undergoing change of life are prone to insomnia and night sweats, often leaving them exhausted, she says.

Dr. Nardone tells patients panicked about memory glitches to practice "sleep hygiene." Be sure the room you sleep in is dark and shielded from noise, so you can sleep beyond 6:00 A.M. Eliminate any stimulating input, she says—no watching TV in bed. Take care not to eat any heavy foods after 7:00 P.M., since vigorous digestion tends to inhibit deep sleep. The same goes for caffeine and chocolate, which can keep you awake.

If restorative rest still eludes you, Dr. Nardone suggests 300 to 500 milligrams of calcium (a glass or two of fat-free milk will do the trick) an hour before bedtime to encourage sleepiness. Or try a small dose of melatonin early in the evening. This sleep-inducing hormone, available in health food stores, also declines with age. Supplements can soothe the body into a deep sleep that is interrupted less often, she says.

whether you're in perimenopause, your doctor should review not only your FSH results but also your medical history and the physical and emotional changes you're experiencing (irregular periods, hot flashes, and so forth).

Menopause: The New View

As baby boomers move through the menopausal arc, attitudes about this transition are changing dramatically. Women whose mothers feared shriveling into inconsequence are celebrating this life passage, proudly declaring themselves crones, goddesses, and menoactivists.

They're at the forefront of the longevity revolution, says Colette Dowling in her book, *Red Hot Mamas: Coming into Our Own at Fifty*. These women are not following the guidelines of past generations but are celebrating the exhilarating possibilities intrinsic in living healthily for decades longer. They are realizing in postmenopause that they have more productive times ahead than they ever thought they would.

"We often hear about the negative impacts of growing older or reaching menopause," says Wulf H. Utian, M.D., Ph.D., executive director of the North American Menopause Society. "Yet when we ask women, we continually hear that they view menopause as the

HONORING MENOPAUSE

"Crone" is the third aspect of the ancient Triple Goddess: Maiden/Mother/Crone. And as more baby boomers reach menopause, croning ceremonies are gaining popularity, says Ann Kreilkamp, Ph.D., of Kelly, Wyoming, founder of the quarterly magazine *Crone Chronicles* and co-founder of Crones Counsel.

Celebrating the crone, as ancient cultures did, means looking beyond appearances and valuing experience, she says. At this point, women enter full maturity, inside and out. "By this new (and very ancient) measure, the crone is the most revered stage of life," she says.

Croning rituals are highly personal events marking what women feel is important about this period of incontrovertible change. They usually involve trusted friends who gather for a meal and act as a protective circle.

Often women recount key life events. Some write songs or chants to explain the new self that emerges from the youth self. Many burn or throw things away to symbolically get rid of ideas they're "done with." These can be anxious musings over a man or images of unrealistic feminine beauty—whatever speaks to you.

One emerging crone wrote her fears about aging on slips of beautiful handmade paper, then hung them on a tree in her home. After 7 days, she and a friend burned their slips of paper, symbolically letting their fears go. "So many people fear the aging process," Dr. Kreilkamp says. "They wanted to celebrate the idea that to become old is a gift."

Another woman gathered friends and read journal entries from the first half of her life. She wanted to commemorate "who I have become out of that past and who I hope and dream to still become."

One budding crone built her ritual around the anthology entitled *When I Am an Old Woman I Shall Wear Purple*. To celebrate the joie de vivre captured by this poem, she dressed in purple, decorated her home with purple flowers and candles, and gave her honored guests ceramic violet pins.

The Order of the Golden Toes is a fun ritual, posted on the Internet by a woman named Metatarsa, who's proud and happy to be deemed a crone. This rite of passage through peri- and postmenopause has two phases: the silver and the gold.

When you realize you're in perimenopause, paint one toenail silver. For every six full moons that pass, award yourself another silver toe. When all 10 toes are silver, you may substitute a gold one every six full moons. (If six moons go by without a period, you may claim a gold toe immediately.) On the momentous occasion of 12 full moons without a period, one large gold toe may be claimed. The second large gold toe may be added after another postmenopausal year.

Metatarsa says that just as only a crone can truly know the inner rewards and golden joys of being a "powerful, untrammeled, and self-directing" woman elder, only she knows about her golden toes—unless, of course, she wears sandals.

beginning of many positive changes in their lives and health." Women surveyed by NAMS said many areas of their lives had improved since menopause—including their family or home lives, sense of personal fulfillment, ability to focus on hobbies or other interests, relationships with their partners, and friendships.

Many of these women credit their positive experiences to the fact that their generation has brought menopause out of the closet, where it's talked about more than in previous generations. Today's women also have better nutritional habits than those of previous generations, as well as a better understanding of menopause in general.

Twenty years ago, few women ever mentioned the word menopause, let alone discussed it with their doctors, friends, or spouses, says Dr. Utian. Today, women have access to a broad range of information on menopause and are very proactive in managing their health as they grow older, he says.

Eight out of 10 women surveyed by NAMS said they would encourage all women to approach the change with an upbeat attitude.

Geraldine, 52, echoes this viewpoint, saying that despite hot flashes, she has a deeper spiritual and positive sense of who she is than when she was younger. "I have plenty of stress and worries, to be sure, but I've learned through experience to do more of what feels good and less of what doesn't," she says. "And I've learned how to access those inner reserves. It's also a huge relief to be much less concerned about how I look and how others are judging me."

Diane, a woman in the midst of the menopause journey, says that while the physical rites of passage are no fun, "in all honesty, I wouldn't trade this stage of life for anything. Over the last 7 years, I've found I'm much more centered, far more confident, happier in my relationship with my husband, and in general, more satisfied with myself as a person. For me, middle age so far has been full of spiritual surprises and a deepening sense of the 'rightness' of me as a woman and a human being."

Patricia Love, Ed.D., a relationship therapist in Austin, Texas, and coauthor of *Hot Monogamy: Essential Steps to More Passionate, Intimate Lovemaking*, says her postmenopausal years have been filled with energy and achievement. Prior to menopause, the hormonal ups and downs of womanhood left her exhausted, she says. Now she's calmer, she doesn't have backaches, and her chronic fatigue is gone. Dr. Love sees herself as the typical postmenopausal woman of the 21st century. Rather than viewing menopause as the start of a long downhill slide, women who actively manage their health are realizing this life passage is simply a "mental pause," says Dr. Love, a time to take stock of what's important to you and then act on it.

"Women get very busy in postmenopause," says Dr. Love, who works with many people in this stage of life. Men are winding down at this age, but women are branching out, trying new things, and starting new careers, she says, noting that postmenopausal women are the fastest growing segment of the entrepreneurial population.

"In so many ways, life for postmenopausal women today is great!" she says.

Or, to quote Margaret Mead, "There is no more creative force in the world than a menopausal woman with zest."

Making the HRT Decision

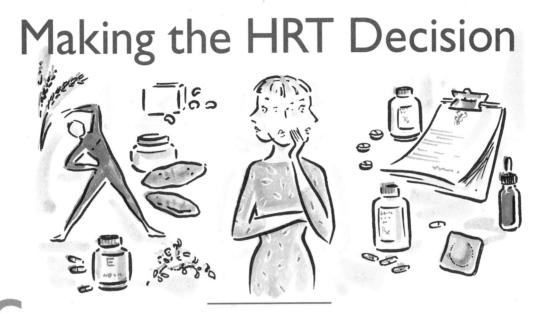

Confused about whether or not to take HRT (hormone replacement therapy)? Know that you're not alone.

"The doctors are confused, so I can't imagine that women aren't," says Machelle M. Seibel, M.D., clinical professor of gynecology and obstetrics at Boston University School of Medicine and a reproductive endocrinologist at The Fertility Center of New England.

Thanks to conflicting studies, confusing reports in the media, and contradictory propaganda, about one-third of all menopausal and postmenopausal women don't know *what* to think about HRT. And with about 50 million of us heading into menopause, plus greater numbers to come, that leaves a lot of us scratching our heads.

When you get through all the research and hoopla, however, it essentially boils down to this: HRT is not the source of all women's evils as its critics say, but neither is it the cure-all others claim.

So to take HRT or not? It's as individual a decision as what color lipstick to buy. Along with your doctor, you need to consider your health, family medical history, risks, and just plain how

you feel about it deep in your gut, says Sharon Youcha, M.D., a gynecologist with a special interest in menopause who is on the clinical faculty at Thomas Jefferson University Hospital in Philadelphia.

The Good and the Bad

Think of the decision to take HRT as a scale: You weigh the benefits on one side, the drawbacks on the other. Whichever side tips the scale determines your decision. But before you start weighing, you've got to know the facts.

The Pros

Bones. The ads might as well say, "Got Estrogen?" For next to calcium, estrogen is probably the biggest ally we have in the quest for strong bones. Basically, it increases growth factors that stimulate bone to grow. So when we lose estrogen in middle age, we begin losing bone. If you take HRT, studies show, that loss slows. One study found that women who took HRT for 5 or more years reduced their risk of

HOW DO THEY MAKE PREMARIN?

The question of the safety and effectiveness of estrogen isn't the only controversy swirling around hormone replacement therapy. How some forms of estrogen are made has people up in arms as well.

The estrogen many doctors prescribe is called conjugated equine estrogen, better known in prescription form as Premarin, one of the most prescribed drugs in the country. The word *equine* provides a hint—Premarin is derived from the urine of pregnant mares. Mares produce high levels of estrogen in their urine until the middle of the third trimester.

On one side of the issue, animal rights activists believe that breeding horses just so the mares can produce estrogen-rich urine is cruel. They also claim that the foals of these pregnant horses are unwanted "by-products."

On the other side are those who feel women shouldn't put a substance such as horse urine into their bodies and that they should be using "natural" or bio-identical estrogens processed from plants.

"Some women view the estrogen in Premarin as an unacceptable choice because it is derived from pregnant mares. But for the majority of women I see, it is a point of interest but not a point of decision making. Would they rather it come from a plant or some other source? Yes. But I don't think that alone is going to stop women from taking estrogen," says Machelle M. Seibel, M.D., clinical professor of gynecology and obstetrics at Boston University School of Medicine and a reproductive endocrinologist at The Fertility Center of New England.

Kwolek, M.D., medical director of the women's health center at the University of Kentucky's Chandler Medical Center in Lexington. Women who take HRT reduce their hot flashes (or power surges, as some of us like to call them) up to 70 percent. For many women, Dr. Youcha adds, HRT is the only way to get through menopause without investing in a towel company. How does it help? One theory is that as estrogen declines during menopause, a chemical called luteinizing hormone (LH) rises, possibly throwing off the way your body's thermostat works. HRT affects the release of that hormone, stabilizing the thermostat like a cool spring day.

Sleep. Estrogen helps you get a better night's sleep. A study conducted in Turku, Finland, found that HRT eliminated the hot flashes, night sweats, and headaches that kept women up at night. Another study at Brown University School of Medicine in Providence, Rhode Island, found HRT helped alleviate sleep apnea, in which you stop breathing several times during the night, in menopausal women. Somehow, researchers speculate, estrogen helps stimulate breathing during sleep.

Mood. It could be the result of getting a better night's sleep, or it could be that HRT actually helps regulate mood, but women on HRT often report feeling less irritable, says Wulf H. Utian, M.D., Ph.D., executive director of the North American Menopause Society in Cleveland.

back and neck fractures 50 to 80 percent, and it's important to continue to take HRT to maintain this benefit. Another series of studies found women taking hormones reduced their risk of hip fractures 25 percent.

Hot flashes. Without question, HRT is the most effective treatment for hot flashes and other perimenopausal symptoms, says Deborah

Memory. The studies aren't completely conclusive yet, but research suggests that estrogen replacement therapy helps improve memory and cognitive function and may even ward off or at least slow the progression of Alzheimer's disease.

Weight. In what may be the greatest incentive to take HRT, researchers at Boston University discovered that women on HRT had significantly less body fat than non-HRT users. A study at Johns Hopkins University in Baltimore found that HRT increased muscle mass while decreasing body fat. Researchers speculate that it's the estrogen drop that contributes to the all-too-common postmenopausal weight gain.

Gum disease. It's bad enough that you probably don't floss enough, but if you're going through menopause, you may be increasing your risk of gum disease in yet another way. Estrogen seems to dampen gum inflammation, thereby slowing the progression of gum disease. A study of 70 women at the University of Nebraska in Lincoln found that those on HRT had less gum inflammation and supporting bone loss than women not taking hormones.

HORMONES THROUGH HISTORY
The Inventors of HRT

Maybe we're the first generation openly talking about taking hormones for health, but we sure aren't the first ones who thought about it. There's evidence that more than 5,000 years ago, Chinese emperors ingested the urine of young women to gain the restorative powers of hormones.

In the modern era, we can thank the research team of Edgar Allen and Edward A. Doisy. They got the ball rolling on the hormone revolution in 1923 with their landmark paper in the *Journal of the American Medical Association*, "An Ovarian Hormone: Preliminary Report on Its Localization, Extraction, and Partial Purification and Action in Test Animals."

The two met and quickly became friends in their medical school library in the early 1920s. So when Dr. Allen wanted to make extracts from ovarian tissue, based on previous research that showed removing the ovaries from rats stopped their estrus cycle (basically, an animal's menstrual cycle), he asked his good friend Dr. Doisy to help. The two set about identifying the hormone that turned out to be estrogen.

As for the progesterone part, they got some help from G. W. Corner and Willard Allen, who identified and explained the role of progesterone in 1927. Then in 1929, Dr. Doisy—continuing his previous estrogen research—actually crystallized estrogen, which was originally called theelin. So by the end of the 1920s, scientists understood and could recreate the roles of both estrogen and progesterone in a woman's body.

Ironically, Dr. Edgar Allen was just 31 and Dr. Doisy only 29 when they published the findings that would later change the science of aging.

The Cons

Blood clots. HRT more than doubles your risk of developing blood clots in your legs, which could dislodge and travel to your lungs (causing a pulmonary embolism) or to your brain (causing a stroke or other serious problems). Oral estrogen elevates blood-clotting factors produced by the liver, which may trigger the formation of blood clots.

Gallstones. HRT also slightly increases your risk of developing gallstones. Because estrogen stimulates the liver to remove cholesterol from the blood and divert it into the gallbladder, gallstones form if too much cholesterol flows into the gallbladder.

Endometrial cancer. Because the additional estrogen stimulates the cells lining your uterus to continue to divide, estrogen replacement therapy alone can increase your risk of this cancer. But that risk is essentially eliminated when progesterone is added to the hormone mix.

Periods. Just when you thought it was safe to throw out the tampons, you start on HRT and begin having periodic vaginal bleeding again. Blame HRT. This is the major reason women stop taking hormones. (Hey, 40 years of periods is more than enough!)

Side effects. Like most drugs, HRT has a laundry list of possible side effects, including severe stomach pain or swelling, pain or numbness in the chest, shortness of breath, severe headaches, changes in vision, and breast lumps. Other, less serious side effects include bloating, breast pain and tenderness, nausea, headaches, and mood swings.

Restrictions. You may not be able to take HRT if you've had breast cancer, liver disease, large uterine fibroids, or endometriosis, because HRT may aggravate these conditions.

The Unknowns

What troubles most of us isn't what we know about HRT—it's what we don't know or at least don't know enough about. The real risk of breast cancer in conjunction with HRT is still up in the

BLAME IT ON HORMONES
Urinary Incontinence

It's only once our bodies stop making estrogen that we realize just how much this single hormone does. Take the bladder, for instance. Estrogen keeps the linings of the bladder and urethra supple and healthy. When we stop making estrogen, our bladder-control muscles weaken, often to the point where a simple sneeze or chuckle can generate an embarrassing accident.

Researchers believe urinary incontinence affects from 30 to 60 percent of all postmenopausal women. But the good news is that it's easily controlled and, better yet, cured, says Rodney Appell, M.D., Scott Professor of Female Urology at Baylor Medical College in Houston.

Hormone replacement therapy is one treatment option for urinary incontinence, but that's not your only choice. With a few simple steps, you can lessen—or perhaps even prevent—this problem.

➤ Add Kegels to your exercise routine. Kegels work the pelvic floor muscles, the same muscles that allow you to control the flow of urine. The great thing about Kegels: You can do them anywhere, and no one has to know. To find these muscles, stop the flow of urine the next time you go to the bathroom—that's the same action you do during Kegels. Quickly contract and relax the muscles

air. Meanwhile, one of the potential benefits of long-term HRT—prevention of heart disease—has been called into question. Here's what we know for sure.

Breast Cancer

Ask any woman considering HRT about her greatest concern and she'll probably tell you: breast cancer. The specter of this dreaded disease looms large over our decision to take hormones. In fact, some experts say it's the number one reason holding most women back.

10 times, then rest for 10 seconds. Then contract again, but this time hold the contraction for 10 seconds or longer. Repeat this two-part process as much as you can, working up to 150 contractions a day. If you're not having success with Kegels, talk with your urologist or gynecologist, says Dr. Appell. Many times, a woman isn't contracting the right muscle. With a quick exam, your doctor can tell you if you're doing it right and help you to correct any technique problems.

- Wear a tampon during exercise, even when you're not menstruating. The tampon puts pressure on the urethra, giving you more urinary control. Take the tampon out as soon as you're done and don't use this as a round-the-clock measure, Dr. Appell warns.

- Go to the bathroom before exercising, even if you don't feel like you need to. The less you have in your bladder, the less likely you are to leak.

- Forget about being a lady—crossing your legs strengthens your pelvic floor muscles. In fact, a study at the University of Utah found that women were nearly 10 times less likely to leak urine if they crossed their legs before they sneezed or laughed.

If these strategies offer no relief, talk to your doctor. There are a variety of treatment options ranging from medication and biofeedback to surgery. "This is a quality-of-life issue—you don't have to just live with it," Dr. Appell says.

"If you could take away the fear of breast cancer, the number of women taking HRT would probably double," says Dr. Seibel. And yet each new study seems to cloud the picture further instead of providing clarity.

As Dr. Seibel says, there's both truth and exaggeration in the information that's presented to us. The key is to put it all in perspective.

First, you need to understand the HRT–breast cancer connection.

A cancer cell forms when the DNA that controls cell division is damaged. By stimulating breast cells to divide, estrogen increases the chance that one of those new cells will have damaged DNA and will then multiply out of control, causing cancer.

Studies show that women who take HRT for 5 years or less—the usual amount of time required to treat menopausal symptoms—probably have little to worry about. There's a very small risk of blood clots.

Questions arise for women who take HRT longer to prevent osteoporosis or heart disease. More than 51 population studies found that the risk of breast cancer increased approximately 30 percent for women who used HRT for 5 years or more. And it's possible that the progesterone added to estrogen replacement therapy to reduce the risk of endometrial cancer actually *increases* the risk of breast cancer.

But before you flush your Premarin down the toilet, consider what these numbers actually mean, a reality that is often lost in the hysterical headlines. Basically, 10 out of every 100 women age 50 and older who have *not* taken HRT or who have taken it for less than 5 years will develop breast cancer— that's the normal breast cancer rate.

Yet out of every 100 women age 50 and older who *have* taken HRT for more than 5 years, 13 or 14 will develop breast cancer. That's 3 to 4 more women per 100.

The bottom line: Taking HRT long term may increase your *personal* risk of developing breast cancer about 4 percent. And keep in mind that while the risk of breast cancer is real, your chances of developing heart disease and osteoporosis are much higher, Dr. Kwolek says.

Future research seeks to clarify the link between HRT and breast cancer, which is still observational and unproven. Until then, you and your doctor have to make decisions based on your history and, obviously, your comfort level. "If you're lying awake at night worrying about breast cancer, then you shouldn't be taking HRT," Dr. Kwolek says.

Heart Disease

For years, many doctors viewed HRT as the ultimate double whammy against osteoporosis and heart disease—two problems that plague women most after menopause.

Years of observational studies backed up this theory by showing that women who took the hormones had fewer heart attacks than those who didn't. Other studies found that women on HRT saw their LDL ("bad") cholesterol level drop about 10 percent, while their beneficial HDL cholesterol increased about 9 percent.

But a 4-year study of 2,700 women, part of the Heart and Estrogen/Progestin Replacement Study (HERS), found in 1998 that women who already had heart disease were 50 percent more likely to have a heart attack during their first 2 years on HRT than those not taking hormones. That risk disappeared by their third and fourth years on hormones, however, with the women having 40 percent *fewer* heart attacks than those taking an inactive substitute. Still, researchers said they wouldn't recommend HRT for women with existing heart disease.

The bottom line: If you have heart disease and are considering HRT for osteoporosis or perimenopausal symptoms, find other treatment options. If you haven't had a heart attack and don't have severe arteriosclerosis, you're probably

WOMEN ASK WHY

Why are there racial and ethnic differences in the use of HRT?

While 12 out of every 100 white women are on HRT (hormone replacement therapy), only 7 out of 100 nonwhite women take the hormones. Researchers point to numerous reasons for the differences.

First, and possibly foremost, most studies looking at the risks and benefits of HRT were conducted with white women. Doctors may be reluctant to recommend HRT to nonwhite women because there is uncertainty about whether the risks and benefits of HRT differ by ethnicity.

Another reason could be differences in how some groups use the health care system. For instance, some research shows that certain ethnic and racial groups are less likely to have health insurance, making it less likely that these women will have a regular physician. Multiple studies have shown that a doctor's recommendation is the primary factor in influencing women to use HRT. Without regular medical care, a woman isn't likely to be given the option of HRT.

Even if women have comparable numbers of medical visits, HRT tends to be prescribed more often to white women

fine taking HRT for your other conditions, Dr. Utian says.

But heart disease prevention shouldn't be the *only* reason you're taking HRT, anyway. The cholesterol benefits you get from hormones are about the same you'd get from a low-fat diet, Dr. Youcha says. And cholesterol-lowering statins and other medications may provide better protection, she says.

Questions to Ask Yourself

Now it's time to put all the pros and cons on the scale. How do you measure it out? Try an-than to black women. Part of this may be that African-American women don't see their gynecologists as often as white women. And it's gynecologists who are more likely to prescribe HRT than other physicians.

There may be more than just race and ethnicity at work, however. Traditionally, women who go on HRT are more affluent and educated than those who don't. Why? These women have easy access to medical care, tend to be healthy, and may be more likely to visit physicians for preventive care.

Another possibility: There may be differences in how certain groups of women view menopause. Some research suggests that African-Americans perceive menopause more as a natural transition than a disorder. This outlook might make them more accepting of their symptoms and less likely to seek medical treatment. Patients with physicians of the same race may be more likely to take HRT.

Expert consulted
Elizabeth Phelan, M.D.
Acting assistant professor of internal medicine
*   and geriatrics*
University of Washington
Seattle

swering these few simple questions, Dr. Utian suggests. Along with your doctor's input and recommendations, your answers will help guide you down the right path.

Do I have perimenopausal symptoms such as hot flashes? If the answer is no, you don't need HRT.

Why do I need HRT? You should not take hormones just because you're a menopausal woman. Your doctor should clearly state why she thinks you need HRT and what your long-term plan of action is.

Do I want to take HRT short term or long term? Women who take HRT simply for menopausal symptoms usually take it for 5 years or less. In that time, there's no increased risk of breast cancer but also no protection from bone loss. If you want to take hormones to ward off osteoporosis, you'll need to take them longer than 5 years, possibly for the rest of your life. For more on osteoporosis and other treatments, see Strong Bones: The Hormonal Connection on page 63.

What does my medical history show? You'll have to go over this with your doctor, but many women either under- or overestimate their own risk of certain diseases. You may fear breast cancer, but your family history and your own bone density may predispose you much, much more to osteoporosis.

Are there other options? Obviously, lifestyle changes make a big difference in the development of heart disease and osteoporosis. And there are other drugs on the market that help treat hot flashes and bone loss. That's not to say these are better than HRT. In fact, you may find HRT is perfect for you. But look at all your other options before deciding.

How do I feel about HRT? Gut feelings go a long way, Dr. Youcha says. If taking HRT seems right medically, but you're stressing out about it, talk to your doctor about the alternatives.

Traveling Down a Different Road

For some women, the answer to the HRT question is a clear no. Whether it's because you can't take HRT—or you just won't—there are plenty of other options that can help you deal with the symptoms of perimenopause and safeguard your health. Here's an A-to-Z guide of various remedies and how they can help you navigate the shoals of menopause.

Remedy: Acupuncture

Best used for: Hot flashes, mood swings

Acupuncture may alleviate many perimenopausal symptoms, including hot flashes, says Beverly Whipple, Ph.D., professor at Rutgers University College of Nursing in Newark, New Jersey. It's thought to work by rebalancing the hormonal system and triggering the release of your brain's feel-good chemicals, endorphins. A Swedish study of 21 women with menopausal hot flashes found that acupuncture significantly reduced their symptoms. Its effects lasted at least 3 months after treatment ended.

Remedy: Black cohosh

Best used for: Hot flashes

The herb black cohosh (*Actea racemosa*) has estrogen-like effects, which enable it to quell hot flashes, Dr. Whipple says. Several clinical trials found that black cohosh reduced hot flashes up to 80 percent. To put your fire out, take 4 milligrams of black cohosh, either in one dose or in two 2-milligram tablets twice a day, but don't use for more than 6 months, says Dr. Whipple.

Remedy: Daily meditation

Best used for: Hot flashes, night sweats, insomnia, prevention of heart disease

Women who practice 15-minute daily meditations experience fewer hot flashes and night sweats and thus sleep better, says Ann Webster, Ph.D., a health psychologist who runs a clinic for perimenopausal and menopausal women at Beth Israel Deaconess Medical Center in Boston. This period of scheduled calm also helps lower blood pressure and relieve stress—two markers for heart disease, she adds. For it to work, you have to make it a habit. Once a day, find a quiet spot where no one will bother you and try this relaxation exercise: Breathe deeply and, with each exhalation, silently repeat a word or phrase. It can be as simple as "relax." Repeat the phrase on each exhalation for 15 minutes. Use this technique when you feel a hot flash coming on.

Remedy: Deep breathing

Best used for: Hot flashes

When you feel yourself heating up, take a deep breath. Deep breathing can reduce hot flashes up to 50 percent, according to studies by Robert R. Freedman, Ph.D., of Wayne State University in Detroit. Slow, deep breathing calms an area of the brain associated with hot flashes. Take six to eight slow, deep, abdominal breaths per minute. Practice for 15 minutes each morning and night and breathe deeply when you feel a hot flash coming on.

Remedy: Flaxseed

Best used for: Hot flashes, vaginal dryness, protection from heart disease

Flaxseed's essential fatty acids act like weak estrogens in your body, helping relieve menopausal symptoms and lubricate vaginal tissues, writes Lana Lew, M.D., an Australian women's health specialist, in her book *The Natural Estrogen Diet*.

They also contain omega-3 fatty acids that help protect your heart. You need 1 to 2 tablespoons of flaxseed a day to get the greatest benefit. Because your body can't absorb the healing properties of the straight seeds, buy ground flaxseeds at health food stores or grind them in a coffee grinder. Then add a tablespoon to your cereal in the morning and another to yogurt, baked goods, or salads to get what you need each day.

Remedy: Layers

Best used for: Hot flashes

Sometimes the flashes are so intense you probably wouldn't care if you stripped down to your bra. But since society isn't too accepting of public nudity, start the day in layers—a tank top covered by a T-shirt covered with a cardigan or jacket. Then, when a flash hits, you can take something off without revealing too much, Dr. Whipple says. When dressing, stick to cotton and other natural fibers as they keep you cooler.

Remedy: Phytoestrogens

Best used for: Hot flashes, prevention of heart disease

With all the talk about using soy to treat perimenopausal symptoms, the benefits of other foods containing valuable phytoestrogens have gotten lost. (For more on soy, check out Soy: Woman-Friendly Hormones from Nature on page 128.) For instance, alfalfa sprouts are a rich source of lignans and coumestans—two estrogen-like plant chemicals. Generously sprinkle sprouts over salads and use on sandwiches. Foods such as black-eyed peas, chickpeas, green peas, lentils, navy beans, red beans, and split peas are other good sources of phytoestrogens. These fiber-rich foods also help ward off heart disease by lowering total and undesirable LDL cholesterol.

Remedy: Sage tea

Best used for: Hot flashes

Long used to treat excessive sweating, the kitchen herb sage can help cool down a hot flash. To make a cup of sage tea, steep 2 teaspoons of dried sage in 1 cup boiled water for 10 to 15 minutes—or add 30 to 60 drops of sage tincture to the water. Use as needed, but only for a short amount of time; prolonged use can actually trigger hot flashes.

HORMONE REPLACEMENT FOR YOUR HUSBAND?

Can't you just picture the commercial? A bunch of guys sitting around watching the big game, drinking a few brews, when one of them pipes up: "Guys, I haven't been feeling myself lately. My doctor thinks I might need to go on HRT. I'm not sure what to do."

A big, burly man named Bud comes back with: "I know how you feel, Al. But since I've been on testosterone, I feel great! I'm vibrant, and my sex life has never been better!"

The guys raise their beer steins in raucous approval, while the name of a prescription flashes on the screen.

It might not be so far-fetched. Male HRT is available now and is expected to grow in popularity in the coming years.

The main hormone in male HRT is testosterone, says Keith Gordon, Ph.D., associate director for reproductive medicine at Organon in West Orange, New Jersey.

As with estrogen in women, testosterone starts to decline during a man's forties. Early on, testosterone deficiency presents itself as general malaise, depression, and perhaps muscle weakness, Dr. Gordon says. As the decline progresses, it can affect sexual function and, in the long term, speed up osteoporosis. To ward off all these troubles, a man can take supplemental testosterone.

But just as with our HRT, he'll have to weigh the benefits against the risks. In his case, supplemental testosterone could bring on benign prostatic hyperplasia, a condition in which the prostate grows larger and pushes against the urethra or bladder, blocking the normal flow of urine. If he has the early stages of prostate cancer, testosterone could also speed the cancer's growth, Dr. Gordon says.

Remedy: Sex

Best used for: Vaginal dryness, hot flashes

Call it Sex R_x. The more you have sex, the healthier and more lubricated your vaginal lining will be. But it gets even better. According to Dr. Whipple, women who have sex at least once a week have twice the level of

IS HRT FOR YOU?

The benefits may outweigh the risks if . . .

❧ You have problematic symptoms of menopause, such as hot flashes, night sweats, mood swings, or vaginal dryness.

❧ You are in natural menopause or experienced surgical menopause through a hysterectomy that removed both of your ovaries.

❧ You have a family history of heart disease or other risk factors, such as high total cholesterol level or low HDL.

❧ You have osteoporosis or a family history of the disease or other risk factors, such as a slight build or low calcium in your diet.

❧ You have a family history of colon cancer.

The risks may outweigh the benefits if . . .

❧ You have active liver or gallbladder disease or severely impaired liver function.

❧ You have a history of blood clots.

❧ You have a personal or family history of breast cancer. (While there is no data to support an increased risk in these cases, your doctor may not think HRT appropriate for you.)

❧ You just intuitively don't feel good about it.

circulating estrogen, which helps relieve hot flashes, too.

Remedy: Vitamin E

Best used for: Hot flashes, heart disease prevention

About 400 international units (IU) of vitamin E a day helps decrease hot flashes by balancing the levels of estrogen in your body. Not only that, but research shows that postmenopausal women who get at least this much vitamin E have a lower risk of death from heart disease. Getting enough vitamin E from a low-fat diet is a bit difficult. So take a vitamin E supplement, no more than 800 IU daily, with a little bit of fat to ensure absorption. Natural vitamin E food sources include nuts, sunflower oil, and wheat germ, says Samantha Heller, R.D., a nutritionist and exercise physiologist at New York University Medical Center.

Remedy: Water

Best used for: Hot flashes, night sweats

Simple cold water can short-circuit or at least reduce the heat of a hot flash, Dr. Whipple says. Try some of these H$_2$O cooldowns:

❧ Keep a bottle of cold water with you at all times. Sip constantly during the day, especially if you feel a flash coming on.

❧ Place an ice cube or a cold pack on your forehead during an episode.

❧ Put cold water in a spray bottle and mist your face when the heat comes on.

Remedy: Water-based lubricant

Best used for: Vaginal dryness

Don't let vaginal dryness keep you and your partner from a good sex life. Water-based lubricants such as K-Y jelly help relieve vaginal dryness, making intercourse easier and less painful, Dr. Whipple says.

Remedy: Walking

Best used for: Osteoporosis, prevention of heart disease, mood swings, depression

Just putting one foot in front of the other will help prevent heart disease and osteoporosis. But it goes beyond that: Walking releases endorphins—those feel-good brain chemicals—so you'll do better emotionally and be less prone to mood swings. To start, try walking at least 30 minutes three to five times a week, Dr. Whipple says.

A study at Hebrew University Medical School in Jerusalem found that adding a bit of running to your walking routine helps build up to three times more bone. If you hate running, take a 60-second jumping jacks break.

Remedy: Writing

Best used for: Mood swings, depression

For some women, their own feelings about menopause trigger mood swings and mild depression. "Many women come in with very negative labels about themselves—they feel they aren't attractive," Dr. Webster says. Instead of trashing yourself, take to pen and paper and write your thoughts down. Then really study them: Are they realistic? Would you say these things about anyone else? Then why say them about yourself? Once these undermining thoughts are on paper, they don't seem so real or overwhelming, Dr. Webster says.

After focusing on your negative thoughts, use writing to shift to the positive. Many women turn menopause into the most powerful time of their lives, since they now have the independence, strength, and experience to accomplish what they want. Write down eight of the most important areas of your life: your family, career, relationships, health, hobbies—whatever you like. Then write down what you want in those areas. Do you want to change careers? Do you want to spend more time with your children? Do you want to start an exercise program? Write these changes down as goals, Dr. Webster says. Just by verbalizing what you want, you'll feel better about yourself.

Remedy: Yoga

Best used for: Mood swings, depression

As part of her natural menopause program, Dr. Webster has women practice yoga to lift their spirits and raise their self-esteem. "We do standing postures that are energizing and empowering—they wake up the body," she says. A great confidence booster is the Warrior Pose. "It makes you feel strong and confident," Dr. Webster says.

Here's how to do it yourself: Standing straight, step forward with one of your legs. Then bend at the knee on the front leg. In the meantime, turn your back foot so it is perpendicular to your front leg. Then raise your hands directly over your head high enough to feel a good stretch in your shoulders. Hold this position for 15 to 30 seconds, then switch to the opposite leg. Strike this pose when you feel down or to start each day full of confidence. For more yoga instruction, check into local classes.

Soy: Woman-Friendly Hormones from Nature

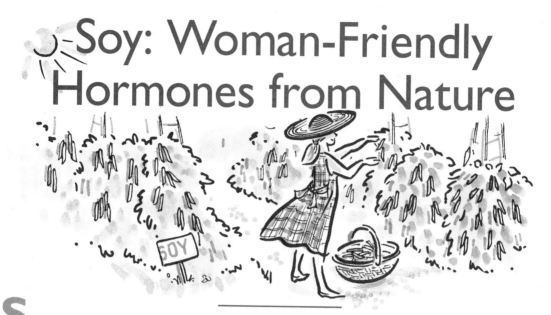

Soybeans—and their sundry variations—have received a lot of press as both a wonder food and a saboteur of health. One week, we hear soy is great, and the next, we're warned against it. What's a health-seeking woman to do?

Practice moderation. While popular opinion trumpets soy as the "next big thing," studies are mostly inconclusive when it comes to *proving* soy's benefits. Nevertheless, scientists do have enough evidence to suggest that at least one serving of soy each day is a pretty good thing. Just don't expect it to cure everything that ails you.

Demystifying That Mysterious Bean

The hype around the soybean concerns compounds called phytochemicals—*phyto* stemming from the Greek work for "plant."

There are thousands of phytochemicals, but the class that gives soy its panache is the phytoestrogens—plant estrogens that mimic our own female sex hormones. By the mid-1990s, scientists had identified more than 300 different plants that contain phytoestrogens, including garlic, wheat, potatoes, cherries, apples, coffee, and, of course, soybeans. Herbs with phytoestrogenic actions include chasteberry (Vitex), black cohosh, and dong quai.

Phytoestrogens are generally considered safe when eaten as part of an ordinary diet, but since they act like hormones, eating too many can alter the way our own hormones function.

These plant estrogens can compete with human estrogens for receptor sites—places on cells that estrogen must latch on to before it can do its job. As a result, they can decrease the amount of strong estrogen (or "bad" estrogen), such as estradiol, that actually latches on to or binds to the sites.

The isoflavones genistein and daidzein, for example, bind to many of the same receptor sites in the breast, uterus, and other areas where estrogen attaches. The idea is that by acting as "antiestrogens," they can then protect these hormonally vulnerable areas from estrogen-stimulated cancers.

But the paradox—and what worries doctors—

is that in addition to blocking estrogens, isoflavones also *stimulate* mild estrogenic activity. This activity can be valuable in women with less available estrogen—such as those in menopause who want the hormone's natural protection for their bones and heart. But it may be troublesome in women who already have enough estrogen, since adding potent isoflavone supplements could raise the total amount of estrogen to unsafe levels.

Test Your Soy Savviness

So before you invest in a refrigerator full of tofu and soy milk, take the quiz below and get the *real* lowdown on soy, your health, and your hormones.

True or False: Soy Is Good for My Cholesterol

True. Heart disease rates for Japanese women are about one-eighth those of women in the United States. Dozens of studies confirm that soy protein lowers levels of LDL ("bad") cholesterol and total cholesterol without affecting HDL ("good") cholesterol.

"The heart-health aspect of soy is the most impressive work on soy so far," says Sadja Greenwood, M.D., assistant clinical professor of obstetrics, gynecology, and reproductive sciences at the University of California Medical Center in San Francisco.

Improving your cholesterol levels lowers your chance of developing high blood pressure or heart disease, which affects 1 in 10 American women ages 45 to 64. Even in women with normal cholesterol levels, soy intake over the years may lower the risk of heart disease. Soy can also reduce the nasty plaque that collects in the carotid artery and, thus, may reduce the risk of stroke, the third leading cause of death for middle-aged and postmenopausal women.

So many studies proved soy protein's heart-healthy benefits that in October 1999, the FDA allowed manufacturers to label soy foods with notices that eating 25 grams of soy protein daily, coupled with a low-fat diet, may reduce the risk of heart disease.

THE UNEXPECTED SOY

Just like the eggs in an Easter egg hunt, soy can turn up where you least expect it.

Take plastic, for example. Jay-lin Jane, Ph.D., professor of food science and human nutrition at Iowa State University in Ames, began developing soy plastic nearly a decade ago. "We were looking for something that could be made from renewable resources, be processed more cleanly, and be more environmentally friendly," she says.

Unlike petroleum-based plastics that require air-polluting solvents for processing and that clog landfills, Dr. Jane's plastics are made from soy protein, water, and other food-grade, nontoxic ingredients. After about 20 days, some of the formulas break down and can be used as an effective crop fertilizer. Other formulas that create a more water-resistant product—say, plastic cups—are more durable, but they're still completely biodegradable. And some formulas are being developed for *edible* products. "It has a natural flavor," she says.

Which puts a whole new spin on the phrase, "Let's dine on plastic tonight."

"We think it's the right direction to work toward solving the pollution problem," Dr. Jane says.

The hidden soy list goes on and on to include nearly everything from fuel and pesticides to paint and waxes—even medical drugs and cosmetics. Who'd have thought this little legume could be so versatile?

SUPER SOY RECIPES

CURRIED TOFU WITH SQUASH AND LIMA BEANS

Try this festive one-dish meal, and your family may like tofu!

1	pound firm tofu, drained
1	tablespoon safflower or canola oil
1½	cups coarsely chopped onion
1½	tablespoons minced fresh ginger
1	teaspoon minced garlic
2½	teaspoons ground coriander
1½	teaspoons whole cumin seeds
1½	teaspoons turmeric
⅛	teaspoon ground red pepper
1	cup vegetable broth or water
¾	teaspoon salt
1	medium butternut squash, peeled, seeded, and cut into ¾" chunks
10	ounces frozen lima beans, thawed
	Ground black pepper
2	cups hot cooked basmati rice

Set the tofu between two plates and place a heavy pot on top. Set aside for 10 minutes to release excess water. Cut into ¾" cubes and set aside.

Warm the oil in a large saucepan over medium-high heat. Add the onion, ginger, garlic, coriander, cumin seeds, turmeric, and red pepper. Sauté for 2 minutes.

Add the broth or water, salt, squash, and tofu. Bring to a boil. Reduce the heat to medium-low, cover, and cook, stirring occasionally, for 15 to 20 minutes, or until the squash is tender.

Mash some of the squash against the sides of the pan to create a thick sauce. Add the beans and stir well. Cover and simmer for 2 to 3 minutes, or until the beans are heated through. Season with the black pepper. Serve over the rice.

Makes 4 servings

Per serving: 464 calories, 14.6 g fat, 11.2 g dietary fiber, 0 mg cholesterol, 486 mg sodium

SPAGHETTI WITH TOFU AND ASIAN SPICES

This tofu dish requires virtually no cooking.

8	ounces spaghetti
⅓	cup creamy peanut butter
2	tablespoons light soy sauce
2	tablespoons mirin (rice wine)
2	tablespoons lime juice
1½	tablespoons dark brown sugar
¼	teaspoon red-pepper flakes
1	red bell pepper, thinly sliced
1	yellow bell pepper, thinly sliced
2	cups coarsely chopped watercress
1	pound silken firm tofu, drained and cut into ½" cubes

Prepare the spaghetti according to the package directions. Drain and set aside.

In a large bowl, mix the peanut butter, soy sauce, mirin, lime juice, brown sugar, and red-pepper flakes.

Add the pasta, red pepper, yellow pepper, and watercress. Toss to coat well. Top with the tofu.

Makes 6 servings

Per serving: 303 calories, 10 g fat, 1 g dietary fiber, 0 mg cholesterol, 567 mg sodium

CLASSIC FRUIT SMOOTHIE

This scrumptious low-fat drink is perfect for breakfast or anytime you get a sugar craving.

1	cup fat-free soy milk
1	cup frozen strawberries
½	frozen banana
1	teaspoon sugar

In a blender, combine the soy milk, strawberries, banana, and sugar. Blend until smooth.

Makes 1 serving

Per serving: 210 calories, 2.4 g fat, 5.8 g dietary fiber, 0 mg cholesterol, 98.6 mg sodium

This health claim is based on soy's *protein* content, stresses Barbara Klein, Ph.D., professor of food science and human nutrition at the University of Illinois in Urbana-Champaign. Because the amount varies among similar types of soy foods, you should read labels carefully. For instance, a glass of plain soy milk has 8 grams of soy protein, whereas vanilla soy milk has just 6 grams.

True or False: Soy Can Ease Menopause Symptoms Just as Effectively as HRT

False, at least at this stage.

It's thought that Asian women experience relatively fewer estrogen-related complaints, such as PMS, hot flashes, and night sweats, than Western women because of their plant-based diets rich in soy. So far, however, clinical studies of soy's effects on hot flashes are contradictory and clinically insignificant. The jury's also still out on whether soy helps vaginal dryness, the other most common menopausal symptom among American women.

Some of the contradictory evidence may be due to the women themselves. "I think people are quite different in their responses," says Dr. Greenwood, who chaired an evidence-based review of the studies on isoflavones as they pertain to menopausal women for the North American Menopause Society (NAMS). "There are those who get relief with soy products and others who don't."

Other researchers note that we couldn't possibly handle the amount of soy protein required to achieve the level of phytoestrogens believed helpful for hot flashes in such studies.

"I can understand why women suffering from hot flashes would want to try soy," says Dr. Greenwood. "I don't see any harm or risk adding soy products regularly to your diet. In my opinion, a serving a day, as in using calcium-fortified soy milk instead of regular milk, is a *perfectly* good thing to do."

True or False: Soy Can Decrease My Risk of Cancer

Possibly. This is an unresolved issue. Because rates of breast cancer are as much as 10 times lower in Asian women than in Western women, researchers surmise that their plant-based diets have a protective effect. Chinese women, for example, are only one-fifth as likely to get breast cancer as American women.

When Asian-American women begin eating like their American-born cousins, however, their cancer risks begin to resemble our own.

Researchers aren't sure exactly *how* soy reduces breast cancer risk—or even if it *is* the soy in the Asian women's diet, which differs in a number of ways from that consumed by the typical American woman. They theorize that isoflavones may reduce the risk by reducing women's own estrogen levels, enhancing the way they process estrogen, or latching on to estrogen receptor sites (thereby preventing their own cancer-enhancing estradiol from binding there).

Genistein, in particular, has attracted a lot of attention. In laboratory test tubes, it can affect cells in two ways: make them multiply (which increases cancer risk) or make them stop multiplying (which decreases risk). Genistein can also block a tumor's blood and nutrient supply, a process called angiogenesis, which halts tumor growth. It also alters or inhibits most types of cancer cell growth in test tubes.

Soy-based products may also have beneficial anticancer effects because isoflavones have strong antioxidant properties. In addition, soybeans contain other phytochemicals—such as saponins, phytates, protease inhibitors, trypsin inhibitors, phytosterols, phenolic acids, and amino acids—which, in the test tube, either slow tumor growth or prevent cancer cells from multiplying.

Soy's protective benefits may also be related to its high fiber content. One cup of cooked soybeans has 7 to 10 grams of fiber. High-fiber diets

I HATE TOFU—WHAT CAN I DO?

With all the alternatives to tofu on the market, you should be able to find an appealing alternative.

There are veggie meats that—unlike their cow counterparts—are low in saturated fat and calories and are cholesterol-free. You can find hot dogs, burgers, bacon, breakfast links, lunch meats, and even chicken salad alternatives—all meat-free. Look closer and you'll discover soy cheeses as well as egg-free egg salad.

But soybeans go beyond imitating animal products. Edamame (eh-dah-MAH-meh) are fresh soybeans. They're high in nutrients and low in fat. Steam them and pop them out of the shell as a snack, a side dish, or an addition to virtually anything requiring a hint of green.

Roasted soy nuts come in flavors like hickory-smoked, barbecue, and Cajun. Or try ones coated in chocolate or yogurt. Sweet or savory, they pack a walloping 78 milligrams of isoflavones in each serving.

Miso, a fermented soy paste, makes a salty soup, sauce, salad dressing, or marinade base. Use it to replace anchovy paste, salt, or soy sauce in recipes. Tamari, a by-product of miso, can be used like soy sauce. (Keep in mind, however, that soybean oil has no isoflavones.)

How about a sweet-tooth satisfier? There's an extensive variety of frozen treats, such as vanilla, chocolate—even Neapolitan—soy-based ice creams. (Keep the gorging under control, though, since a half-cup of these treats has only about 1 or 2 grams of soy protein.)

Try soy nut butter in place of peanut butter for a lower-fat alternative. In your favorite recipes, use soy butter instead of regular, substitute one-fourth of the required flour with soy flour, or replace all the milk with soy milk or silken tofu.

If you don't like the flavor of soy in commercial drinks or desserts, mask the taste with a splash of almond extract. Or add fat-free chocolate syrup.

Also look in your cereal aisle for recent soy additions.

If you're allergic to soy, there are still some alternatives for getting your daily isoflavone counts. Try fava beans, raw clover sprouts, granola bars, split peas, and the spice fenugreek, washing any of it down with a cup of Japanese green tea.

have been linked to a lower incidence of breast cancer because fiber helps rid the body of estrogens that can lead to cancer. Further, women who have diets high in soy isoflavones have longer menstrual cycles, so they have fewer cycles overall. The fewer menstrual cycles, the lower the breast cancer risk.

Additionally, several studies suggest that soy phytoestrogens may stop or slow the growth of cells in the uterine lining, a risk for cancer of the uterus that is associated with taking synthetic estrogen.

True or False: Soy Can Protect My Memory

True. "We know that soy can help protect against age-related memory decline," says Helen Kim, Ph.D., research associate professor at the University of Alabama in Birmingham. "But there's no evidence that it *improves* memory."

In one study conducted at Wake Forest University School of Medicine in Winston-Salem, North Carolina, rats put into menopause were given varying doses of soy phytoestrogens, estradiol, and combinations of the two before they were set loose in a familiar maze. The rats getting the phytoestrogens remembered their way through the maze better than those who didn't get them.

But there are relatively few studies on humans. In fact, in a report from the Honolulu-Asia Aging Study, middle-aged men in Hawaii showed an apparent increased risk of dementia and memory loss if they ate at least two servings of tofu a week—but the researchers couldn't prove that it was actually the *tofu* that did the damage.

The results could be due to the Asian lifestyle, suggests Dr. Kim. For example, her grandmother, who came to the United States from Korea, lived in a traditional way, in which the family waited on her. Thus, older people can become sedentary and have little mental stimulation. As a result, they are at higher risk for memory decline.

True or False: Soy Can Lower My Risk of Osteoporosis

True. Certainly, being female, menopausal, and sedentary increases your risk of developing osteoporosis, which affects nearly 8 million American women. (See Strong Bones: The Hormonal Connection on page 63 for more.) But a low-calcium diet also increases your risk. And the more animal protein you eat, the less calcium you absorb. Soy foods not only provide additional calcium but also are an excellent source of nonanimal protein.

Just 1 cup of cooked soybeans has 175 milligrams of calcium (more than 94 milligrams of isoflavones). One serving of tofu has about 400 milligrams of calcium (about 30 milligrams of isoflavones). And 1 cup of fortified soy milk has nearly 10 percent of the recommended daily allowance for calcium (and up to 24 milligrams of isoflavones).

Soy isoflavones also appear to increase bone mass in postmenopausal women. One study found that postmenopausal women who ate isolated soy protein containing 90 milligrams a day of isoflavones for 6 months significantly increased the bone density in their lower spines and helped prevent dowager's hump.

Researchers suspect a minimum of 50 milligrams of isoflavones—the amount in 25 grams of soy protein—a day may improve bone health.

True or False: Soy Can Decrease Pain

True. Scientists sort of stumbled upon this one when they noticed that some groups of rats had less pain than expected following surgery. The rats ate a diet of 20 percent soy protein before and after the surgery. The less soy the rats ate, the less pain protection they had.

The researchers aren't sure why soy—particularly its phytoestrogens—has this numbing effect, and they aren't certain similar effects would appear in humans, but the future could hold soy-based foods as presurgery pain reducers.

True or False: I Can Rely on Tofu for My Dietary Isoflavones

False. Not all soy products are created equal. How they're processed and where they're grown affect their isoflavone content, and some processes remove almost all the phytochemicals. Even the way the isoflavones are isolated can alter their effects.

If you're thinking of adding more soy to your diet, do it gradually, recommends Dr. Klein. "Don't suddenly have four glasses of soy milk, tofu at each meal, and some soybeans in the afternoon. You're going to find yourself feeling uncomfortable," she advises. Soy is a bean, after all. And because soybeans contain more indigestible carbohydrate than other beans, they have a greater potential to turn us into human Hindenburgs. "Americans who want to hop on the soy bandwagon forget that Asians have been consuming soy products since they were infants. Their metabolic systems are set up to deal with soy."

True or False: Isoflavone Supplements Are Just as Effective as Soy Foods

False. Although these supplements do contain the plant versions of estrogens, isoflavone concen-

JUST WHAT *IS* TOFU, ANYWAY?

"Bean curd" is made in much the same way as cheese. Soaked soybeans are cooked into a milky solution and filtered through a cloth. The resulting curds are pressed into cakes. These sponge-like, tasteless bricks take on the flavor of whatever they're mixed with in a variety of dishes, from smoothies to omelets and lasagna. But the many varieties of tofu could confuse even the most skillful cook.

- Silken tofu is smooth—almost creamy—and can be added to salad dressings, milk shakes, sauces, and most anything that's pureed or blended.
- Soft tofu is good for mashing and scrambling.
- Firm or extra-firm tofu is great for slicing, dicing, and crumbling.

But don't stop at tofu. Tempeh (TEM-pay) is a form of fermented soybeans that's slightly more flavorful—and meat-like—than tofu. Grill it on shish kebabs, stir-fry it with veggies, and use it in a variety of ways similar to firm tofu. You can also reduce the amount of meat in a dish by adding tofu or tempeh to "stretch" out the meat.

Then there's soy protein isolate (or isolated soy protein). Soybeans are ground, and the fat, sugars, and carbohydrates removed, leaving nearly pure protein in flake or powder form. It's easily digestible and contains isoflavones as well as other phytochemicals. You can add it to anything from juice to dessert; try a scoopful in soup or macaroni and cheese. But watch the amount. Just 1 ounce could contain 23 grams of soy protein.

---

trations aren't standardized, nor does the United States regulate their content.

Studies analyzing random batches of different isoflavone preparations show that, even within the same brands, there are variations in the amount of isoflavones they contain, says Dr. Kim.

And isoflavones extracted from soy haven't been shown to lower cholesterol.

Supplements also have the potential to be overused, explains Dr. Greenwood. "We don't know enough about the long-term effects of supplements. I'm not in favor of them."

Thus, opt for whole foods rather than supplements. Asian women get anywhere from 30 to 80 milligrams of isoflavones daily from soy foods.

True or False: Soybeans Have a Lot of Fat

True, but they are low in saturated fat and are cholesterol-free. They are also high in omega-3 fatty acids, which alone may prevent severe menstrual cramps, macular degeneration, fatal heart attacks, depression, and maybe even breast cancer.

Tofu is also low in calories (about 45 to 55 calories per 3-ounce serving), but about half of those calories come from unsaturated fat. There are lighter forms of tofu, though, which lowers the fat content to about 2.1 grams per 3 ounces. Soy also has a host of other essential vitamins and minerals, such as calcium, phosphorus, iron, magnesium, thiamin, riboflavin, and niacin. And tempeh adds vitamin B_{12} to this potpourri of nutrients.

So, How Savvy Are You?

- 8 or more correct: Soy superstar
- 6–7: Pretty impressive
- 4–5: Appropriately aware
- 2–3: Not much of a news follower
- 0–1: What's a soybean?

PART THREE

Odds
You Can
Beat

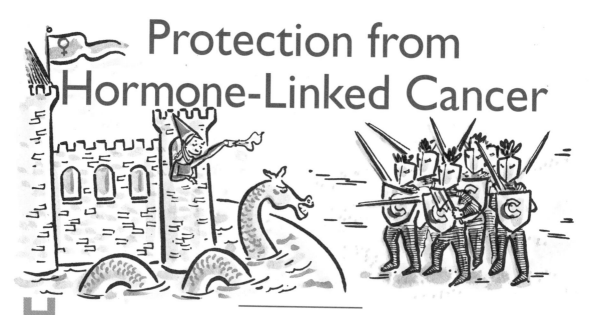

Protection from Hormone-Linked Cancer

Here's the bad news: By virtue of being human, we're all at risk for cancer. No disease-free family tree or model lifestyle can exempt us. Deep in our DNA, something goes wrong (possibly because of too much sunlight, tobacco, or radiation), a normal gene changes into a cancer gene, it gets turned on, and our immune systems don't catch it.

But here's the good news: How we live seems to have nearly as much influence on our cancer risk as our genetic makeup. So there are things we can do to make "the big C" more of a "lowercase c." We can be aware of family risks (such as a mother with cancer), reduce our exposure to cancer-causing toxins (such as chemicals or cigarette smoke), and try to boost an immune system that isn't up to par. We can also get regular screenings to catch cancers when they're small and thus more curable.

And the good *and* bad news? Our hormones can help or hurt the situation. For example, stress hormones may increase our risk of cancer, but progesterone may protect us against some cancers. Here's how to take what researchers know so far and put it to work for you.

Stress and Cancer

That tooth-grinding tension you feel when you're stressed may be just the fin skimming the surface of the water. Underneath, there may be a giant stress shark chomping away at your health.

"I think stress contributes to either cancer or a poor outcome from cancer," says M. Michelle Blackwood, M.D., breast surgeon at the Blackwood Breast Center in Stamford, Connecticut.

Normally, when your immune system identifies an odd-looking invader (like a cancer cell), it wastes no time attacking it. But when big stresses hit, like an overbearing mother, a lost job, or a cancer diagnosis, a series of reactions occurs: Levels of the stress hormones adrenaline and cortisol rise; they intoxicate your immune cells, rendering them less competent. So instead of attacking mutant invader cells, the immune cells swoon and allow these invaders to wreak havoc.

"In short, the link between stress and cancer may be related to suppression of the immune system," says Beth Karlan, M.D., director of gynecologic oncology at the Gynecologic Cancer Foundation and director of the Gilda Radner Ovarian Cancer Program in Los Angeles.

And if you're the type to always make nice when you really want to rage at the world—what's called a type C—you may be raising your cancer risk even more. When you submerge your anger, your cortisol just festers, increasing your vulnerability to cancer.

The good news: There are actions you can take to reduce your stress level and, therefore, lower your cancer risk. For dozens of stress-relieving tips, see Fight or Flight: The Stress Hormones on page 52.

Endometrial Cancer

Endometrial cancer—cancer of the lining of the uterus—is the most common reproductive cancer in women. About 36,000 women are diagnosed per year.

Before menopause, the endometrium grows each month in response to estrogen and progesterone, preparing the uterus for a fetus. When you don't get pregnant, it's sloughed off and expelled during your period.

After menopause, your uterus literally lies down and relaxes. In the process, it deflates and flattens out like a pancake. But the endometrial cells are still in there, and with maturity, they become more vulnerable to cancer.

Estrogen replacement therapy ups the risk, because too much estrogen gets the endometrium growing again. The more growth

> ### CANCER WARNING SIGNS
>
> See your doctor if you experience any of the following symptoms.
>
> **Endometrial Cancer**
> - Abnormal bleeding or spotting
> - Pelvic pain
>
> **Breast Cancer**
> - A lump in your breast
> - Thickening, swelling, or distortion in your breast
> - Unusual breast tenderness
> - Skin irritation or dimpling of breast skin
> - Nipple pain, scaliness, or retraction
>
> **Ovarian Cancer**
> - Enlarged abdomen
> - Persistent digestive discomfort that cannot be explained by any other cause
> - Rarely, vaginal bleeding
>
> **Lung Cancer**
> - Persistent cough
> - Blood in sputum (mucus)
> - Chest pain
> - Recurring pneumonia or bronchitis
>
> **Skin Cancer**
> - Change in the size or color of a mole
> - Scaliness, oozing, or bleeding of a bump or nodule
> - Spread of pigmentation beyond its border
> - Itchiness, tenderness, or pain

and the more cells there are, the higher the likelihood that one will turn cancerous.

That's why most hormone replacement therapy (HRT) includes progesterone with the estrogen. Progesterone helps protect against endometrial cancer by calming down the estrogen-stimulated cells.

But there are things you can do beyond HRT to reduce your risk of endometrial cancer.

Investigate abnormal bleeding. "If you're over 55 and you no longer get your period, *any* vaginal bleeding is abnormal," says Donna Sweet, M.D., professor of internal medicine at the University of Kansas School of Medicine in Wichita. If you're bleeding irregularly and you're pre- or perimenopausal, talk to your doctor. It could be something simple, like fibroids. And even if it turns out to be endometrial cancer, it's very treatable if caught early.

Eat isoflavones. Found in soy products, isoflavones seem to balance the estrogen effects and keep estrogen levels out of the danger zone.

Control your weight. "Fat is an endocrine organ that makes estrogen-like hormones," says Dr. Karlan. Just 30 extra pounds make you three times more likely to get endometrial cancer, and 50 extra pounds increase your risk tenfold.

WOMAN TO WOMAN
She Found a Lump

At 48, Helene Kosakowski of Reading, Pennsylvania, felt very tired. Then one day she found a lump in her breast. It turned out to be estrogen-sensitive breast cancer.

I never did routine checks on my breasts. I was a nurse, and I taught other women to do them, but I never performed them on myself. I didn't think it could happen to me.

When I did find a lump, I went immediately to my family doctor. He sent me for a mammogram that day.

When they repeated the mammogram a few times, I knew something was wrong. Being a nurse, I wasn't about to leave without talking to the radiologist, so I was able to look at my film that day. The lump looked like a small sphere. It had finger-like protrusions, so I knew it had spread. I made an appointment with a surgeon for the following week, and I left for a Disney World vacation.

Needless to say, I was panicked throughout the weeklong vacation. I still had some hope that it wasn't cancer. When I returned, the surgeon killed my hope—it was cancer. And from the biopsy, he could tell the tumor was estrogen-sensitive, meaning the cancer cells were using estrogen to grow. He scheduled my surgery—a lumpectomy (removal of the tumor) and a partial mastectomy (removal of part of my breast)—for March 7, my birthday.

Breast Cancer

With all the races, pink ribbons, and celebrities talking about their breast cancer, it's a hard disease to ignore. And we shouldn't ignore all the hype, because close to 183,000 women get breast cancer each year.

Although estrogen is considered a key player in breast cancer—both its advent and its progress—there are two schools of thought on how much of a role it actually plays.

Some research suggests estrogen may do to our breast cells what too many desserts do to our fat cells—make them grow and divide. And if any of the breast cells are already cancerous, estrogen feeds their growth. The other school disagrees and sees estrogen as more protective than causative in breast cancer development. If you do develop breast cancer while on estrogen, it will typically be a type that is more easily treated.

Unfortunately, passing the menopause mile-

Then, in April, I had a modified radical mastectomy (removal of my entire breast) and an axillary dissection (removal of some of my lymph nodes) because the cancer had spread. I chose not to have breast reconstruction. Instead, I wear a prosthesis.

Six months of chemotherapy followed. Emotionally, this was a scary time. Every day, I just got up and tried to make things as normal as possible. I drove myself to chemo. It was still business as usual. If I went on social outings or traveled with my husband, I simply put on a scarf and a hat and dressed myself up.

After my chemotherapy was complete, I started taking tamoxifen (Nolvadex), and I have been taking it since. Tamoxifen stops estrogen from being produced in my body, so the hormone can't feed the cancer. Tamoxifen has its downside; it brings on hot flashes, weight gain, and the fear of endometrial cancer. My treatment is to end in October 2001.

Today, at age 52, I'm doing well. I devote a lot of time volunteering with the American Cancer Society, helping women who are going through the same thing I did.

If I can give any advice to women going through a bout with breast cancer, it's that you have choices. You don't have to have a breast reconstruction. I never had one. I look good and have a nice body, except I'm missing a breast and wear a prosthesis. It's your body, and you need to look at all the options before you make a decision.

stone doesn't seem to lower your chances of estrogen-positive breast cancer.

The older you get, the greater your chances of getting breast cancer. One reason may be that although your ovaries no longer make estrogen after menopause, there's still enough estrogen hanging around in your tissues to stimulate the growth of breast cancer.

Yet, despite the various theories, estrogen replacement therapy has not been *proven* to increase breast cancer risk. "In fact, most breast cancer cases occur in women who are post-menopausal and have never been on hormone replacement therapy," says Dr. Blackwood.

Another theory suggests that we get more breast cancer as we age because of the overall deterioration our bodies undergo, not because of the estrogen. "We're at the highest risk of breast cancer when we have the *least* amount of estrogen in our bodies," says Dr. Blackwood.

Progesterone also causes cells to divide in the breasts, says Malcolm Pike, Ph.D., professor in the department of preventive medicine at the University of Southern California in Los Angeles. A study conducted at screening centers throughout the United States looked at 46,355 postmenopausal women who had used HRT in the previous 4 years and found that those who took estrogen replacement therapy alone increased their risk of breast cancer by 1 percent each year. Those who took an estrogen/progesterone combination increased their risk *8 percent* each year.

Testosterone may also play a part. Women with breast cancer have 30 to 100 percent more testosterone than healthy women. It's not known exactly what testosterone does in breast tissue to increase the risk. One theory suggests that it stimulates breast cells to grow and divide, increasing the odds that the cancer switch will turn on in one of those cells.

Hormones also play a role once the cancer has developed. Some breast cancers have receptors for estrogen or progesterone, sometimes referred to as ER-positive and PR-positive. On the one hand, it's good to have a hormone-sensitive

Should I take tamoxifen as a breast cancer preventive?

Tamoxifen (Nolvadex) is a great treatment for the majority of breast cancers, especially estrogen-sensitive ones. But doctors hesitate to prescribe it to *prevent* breast cancer because it can increase the risk for endometrial cancer. So before you decide to take tamoxifen as a preventive measure, you should examine the pros and cons.

One good reason to take tamoxifen is if you're genetically at risk for the disease. Then your risk of getting breast cancer is higher than your risk of getting endometrial cancer from the drug. If you still have your uterus, doctors will carefully monitor you with ultrasound for any signs of endometrial cancer and any endometrial thickening. They'll do occasional biopsies to look for any tissue changes. If you've had a hysterectomy, you don't have to worry at all about endometrial cancer.

Obesity seems to make the effects of tamoxifen on the endometrium worse. In postmenopausal women, a reaction can occur in body fat that actually creates the most potent form of estrogen—estradiol—which can feed endometrial cancer cells. So if you're overweight, you should give tamoxifen careful thought and talk to your doctor about your options.

Another catalyst for endometrial cancer is estrogen replacement therapy (ERT). If you're on ERT, you're already at an added risk for endometrial cancer. So the tamoxifen may be the straw to break the camel's back. Make sure you discuss this with your doctor.

Experts consulted

Leslie Bernstein, Ph.D.
Chair of cancer research and professor of
    preventive medicine
Keck School of Medicine
University of Southern California
Los Angeles

Donna Sweet, M.D.
Professor of internal medicine
University of Kansas School of Medicine
Wichita

tumor, because it's more likely to respond to hormone-blocking drugs like tamoxifen (Nolvadex). On the other hand, ER- or PR-positive breast cancer is fueled by estrogen or progesterone, so you have to be extra careful to avoid exposure to those hormones.

There are things you can do to reduce your overall risk of breast cancer.

Get a mammogram. Unless the First Lady invites you to lunch on the day you've scheduled a mammogram, keep your appointment. "Get a mammogram every 1 to 2 years after age 40. If you have a mother or sister with breast cancer, get one every year from age 35 on," says Dr. Sweet. "Early detection can really make a difference in the long-term outcome."

Slim down. More fat equals more unopposed estrogen (estrogen without a progesterone parent keeping it under control), which increases your risk of breast cancer. So a lean body means less estrogen and a lower risk of breast cancer.

Take your breasts for a walk. A study conducted at the University of Southern California School of Medicine showed that women who exercised at least 4 hours per week for at least 12 years and didn't gain much weight in adulthood were 29 percent less likely to get breast cancer than women who never exercised at that level.

Make it a virgin daiquiri. Your arteries may feel pretty good after a few drinks, but your breasts have a low tolerance. A combined analysis of more than 50 studies found that as few as two alcoholic drinks a day can increase your breast cancer risk by 25 percent, no matter if you drink cheap vodka or a fine red wine.

Ovarian Cancer

Ovarian cancer is the most frightening female cancer because it usually yields no symptoms until the disease is far along in development. Many women don't know they have it until the tumor is so large they look pregnant or until it pushes on the bladder or intestines and causes urinary problems or constipation.

Yet it is second only to endometrial cancer as the most common reproductive cancer in women, with about 23,000 new cases diagnosed each year.

A family history of ovarian cancer is the biggest risk factor for the disease, so there aren't a lot of hands-on things you can do to reduce your risk. If you have a mother, sister, grandmother, aunt, or daughter who had ovarian cancer, your risk is higher, especially if your relative got it at an early age.

It seems that a mutated gene (possibly BRCA 1 or 2) is to blame in some cases. If ovarian cancer appears on one of your family tree branches (from either your mother's or your father's side), talk to your doctor about your options. If you're overweight, she might suggest you take off some pounds, since obesity is an added risk factor. She may suggest you take birth control pills, which seem to help prevent ovarian cancer, even in women at risk.

Your hormonal history can also positively or negatively affect your risk of ovarian cancer. For example, women with polycystic ovary syndrome (PCOS), who don't ovulate normally, have an increased risk for ovarian cancer. "There's something funky about these ovaries that keeps them from ovulating," says Dr. Karlan. "So it could be the lack of *normal* ovulation and hormone pro-

duction that increases the risk of ovarian cancer in these cases." But this is just a theory.

Women with PCOS also have higher levels of male hormones like testosterone, which might also play a role in ovarian cancer. "But this, too, needs further study," says Dr. Karlan.

Additionally, every pregnancy could reduce your risk. Researchers aren't quite sure why. And this pregnancy link may be genetic—some women are protected by pregnancy hormones and the subsequent suppression of ovulation they bring; others aren't. "The mechanisms behind this genetic link haven't been worked out yet," says Dr. Karlan.

Birth control pills are also protective, possibly because they, like pregnancy, stop ovulation or have other hormonal effects on the ovary. A study conducted at the Women's College Hospital of the University of Toronto and reported in the *New England Journal of Medicine* looked at pairs of sisters who had the BRCA 1 and 2 genes. In each pair, one got ovarian cancer, and one didn't. Even in these high-risk families, those taking birth control pills were 50 percent less likely to get the cancer. "It has been long known that birth control pills significantly reduce a woman's risk of ovarian cancer and that risk reduction is related to how long she has taken the Pill," says Dr. Karlan.

It could also be the *progestin* (the artificial form of progesterone) in the birth control pills that helps. "There's some animal data suggesting that progestin makes ovaries shed their surface cells early, so cells don't hang around long enough to become cancerous," says Dr. Karlan.

If you aren't a smoker, you can take birth control pills as long as you want. It's the total number of years you're on the Pill between your first and last periods that's important. So if you take it for 3 years in college, 4 years in your thirties, and 3 years in your forties, you'll have 10 total "Pill years" under your belt.

A study conducted at the University of Pittsburgh found that women who regularly exercised—participating in activities like swimming, hiking, and skating—reduced their risk of ovarian cancer 27 percent compared with less active women. One reason, the researchers speculate, may be that physically active women tend to ovulate less often and thus generate more tumor-suppressing hormones and fewer tumor-promoting hormones.

Once ovarian cancer develops, it seems to grow independent of hormones, Dr. Karlan says. Unlike endometrial and breast cells, ovarian cells don't house estrogen receptors, so estrogen doesn't fuel cancer in ovaries like it does in the endometrium and the breast.

Lung Cancer

About 48,000 women are diagnosed with lung cancer each year—about one-quarter the number of new breast cancer patients. But more women *die* of lung cancer than any other cancer, because lung cancer is very difficult to treat.

And it's not just cigarettes that are to blame. Simply being female may increase your lung cancer risk.

A study at the University of Pittsburgh found that lung cancer cells contain more estrogen receptors than normal cells, suggesting that lung cancer is vulnerable to estrogen.

So we may be at a higher risk than our husbands, whether we carry cigarettes in our purses or not. And if we do light up, we're 20 to 70 percent more likely to get lung cancer than men who smoke. "We're not sure whether smoking has anything to do with the presence of the estrogen receptors," says Jill Siegfried, Ph.D., vice-chairperson of the department of pharmacology at the University of Pittsburgh and author of the study. "We have a little data suggesting that long-term smokers have more estrogen receptors than nonsmokers, but we need to do a larger study to verify that."

The good news: Lung cancer is one of the most preventable forms of cancer, because the primary cause is known. Cigarettes cause more than 80 percent of lung cancer cases, so the most crucial prevention tactic is clear: Don't smoke.

If you don't smoke, you can reduce your risk by ducking clouds of secondhand smoke and steering clear of cancer-causing chemicals like asbestos, air pollution, and radon.

Skin Cancer

Some women ignore warnings about the ozone layer and lethal sun rays, basking with no worries of future wrinkles. Others are more cautious and regularly comb their skin for moles that may have changed since last week. If you're the latter, give yourself a gold star.

An estimated 1.3 million people are diagnosed each year with the less serious forms of skin cancer, called basal cell carcinoma and squamous cell carcinoma. Another 47,700 are diagnosed with the most serious malignant melanomas each year. So when it comes to skin cancer, you can't be too careful, especially if you're pregnant, taking hormone replacement therapy, or on birth control pills, because estrogen increases the odds that a mole will turn shady.

In a study conducted in Korea and published in the *Journal of the Academy of Dermatology*, researchers watched a woman's birthmark throughout her pregnancy. The mark grew bigger and more tender during pregnancy, only to return to normal once she gave birth. It seems that estrogen, which rises during pregnancy, affected the birthmark.

"Hormones help control the pigmentation of our skin," explains Debra Jaliman, M.D., clinical instructor of dermatology at the Mount Sinai School of Medicine in New York City. Hormones won't create a new mole, but they may cause one to suddenly go bad.

It works like this: You're lounging in the sun with your SPF 25 tanning

THE WISE STUDY

Both hormone replacement therapy (HRT) and birth control pills may increase a woman's risk for breast and endometrial cancers. Now, researchers on the Women's Insights and Shared Experiences (WISE) study want to find out how these hormones interact with genetic mutations and other environmental exposures to cause breast cancer.

"We are primarily interested in the interaction of HRT or birth control pills and a woman's genetic makeup," says Timothy Rebbeck, Ph.D., associate professor of epidemiology at the University of Pennsylvania School of Medicine in Philadelphia and co-principal investigator on the study. The researchers will specifically look at the genes related to estrogen or progesterone metabolism.

The results could eventually help pinpoint women who may be at an increased risk of breast and endometrial cancers if they take these hormones, says Brian Strom, M.D., professor of biostatistics and epidemiology and professor of medicine at the University of Pennsylvania School of Medicine, who is principal investigator on the study.

The portion of the WISE study related to breast cancer involves 3,200 women over age 50, and the endometrial cancer portion involves 2,000 women of all ages. Cancer patients and women without cancer are randomly chosen throughout the Philadelphia area and interviewed over the phone. Researchers also review their medical histories and collect DNA samples.

So far, preliminary data from the study indicates that our genes do indeed work together with our environment to help determine our risk of breast or endometrial cancer. "There are a lot of directions our research may take us; but we hope ultimately that the research will help us develop improved methods of cancer prevention," says Dr. Rebbeck.

WISE started in November 1998. It's funded for 5 years, but the researchers suspect it may continue and expand beyond that time.

oil. The cells in a mole get hot and bothered, and they start to morph into melanoma cancer cells. Estrogen may help this transformation from good cell to bad by rushing to the melanoma cells, hopping onto the estrogen receptors that live on them, and feeding the bad cells so they can grow.

Estrogen also seems to have a partner in crime when it comes to melanomas: progesterone. "Progesterone may cause the pigmentation to spread," says Dr. Jaliman. So estrogen feeds the bad cells, and progesterone helps them migrate to other body areas.

And when estrogen goes to work on a mole, it doesn't beat around the bush. It increases your risk of the *worst* kind of skin cancer, malignant melanoma. Ironically, it doesn't seem to fuel the less harmful basal cell and squamous cell carcinomas, says Dr. Jaliman. These less serious forms look like pink nodules or red scaly patches, whereas malignant melanomas look more bizarre. They show up as a dark brown or black mole with irregular borders and colors— usually shades of blue/black, red, or white. They most often appear on the upper back or lower

legs, but they can also pop up on other parts of your body.

Risk factors for skin cancer include:

- Being blond with light skin and blue or green eyes
- Having red hair
- Having freckled skin
- Early blistering or sunburn before the age of 18
- A family history of skin cancer
- Having more than 50 moles on your body

Of course, sun exposure also plays a big part, so here are some of Dr. Jaliman's suggestions on staying shaded.

- Keep out of the sun between 10:00 A.M. and 3:00 P.M.
- Wear a hat with a 2-inch brim to keep the sun off your face.
- Seek a tree or awning for shade.
- Wear long sleeves and long pants or skirts, when feasible.
- *Always* use sunscreen with an SPF (sun protection factor) of at least 15 that contains micronized zinc oxide and reapply it every 2 hours and after swimming or sweating.

Take Steps against Environmental Hormones

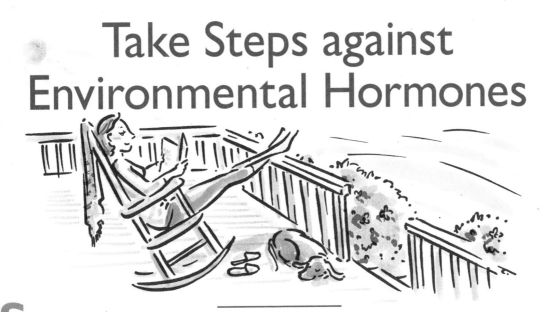

Something has happened to the fish in Great Britain and the United States. To the alligators and red-eared turtles in Florida's Lake Apopka. To the gulls in the Puget Sound region of Washington state and to the gulls and terns of the Great Lakes region of Michigan.

Something that has altered their hormone levels, affected their fertility, caused reproductive tract cancers, and deformed their offspring.

Evidence points to chemicals in our water, air, and soil as the likely cause of these problems. These chemicals, called hormonally active agents (HAAs), pass from female birds, fish, and reptiles to their offspring, affecting their sexual and reproductive development.

Some doctors and scientists are concerned that HAAs may also be affecting human health—not only ours but the health of our children, great-grandchildren, and great-great-grandchildren.

Of the more than 70,000 synthetic chemicals used today, only a fraction have been adequately studied for toxic effects in people, says Ted Schettler, M.D., of Boston, science director of the Science and Environmental Health Network and coauthor of *Generations at Risk: Reproductive Health and the Environment.*

"In addition, we have very limited information about actual human exposures to many synthetic chemicals," says Dr. Schettler. Whether HAAs threaten human health—and, if so, to what degree—is fraught with controversy. According to some scientists, there's no evidence that the levels of HAAs to which we're exposed cause health effects.

Others disagree, believing that the health effects of HAAs may not be apparent for years—or for generations. But there are things you can do to protect yourself.

Weighing the Evidence

Used in pesticides, plastics, household products, and industrial chemicals, HAAs (also called endocrine disrupters) affect hormones in a variety of ways. They "impersonate" female sex hormones (estrogens) or male sex hormones (androgens), block their effects, or otherwise interfere with normal hormonal activity.

But while studies of animals, humans, and

cells offer compelling evidence that high concentrations of HAAs cause serious reproductive and developmental problems, experts don't yet know how lower amounts—those we're typically exposed to every day—affect our health.

Because many act like natural estrogens, however, it's likely that any problems would be related to sexual development, reproduction, and cancers of the breasts and reproductive organs. What's worrisome is that, in the past several decades, the United States and other countries have experienced a rise in the rates of breast, prostate, ovarian, and testicular cancer—all of which are fueled by estrogen.

Further, during the 1970s and 1980s, the number of boys born with hypospadias, an abnormality of the penis, doubled in the United States. Finally, one large study suggests that, worldwide, there has been a substantial decline in the quality of male semen over the past 50 years. This controversial finding has fueled intense debate in the general population.

As has much of the research on HAAs.

Right now, "the field of endocrine disruption resembles an unfinished jigsaw puzzle," says Gina Solomon, M.D., assistant clinical professor of medicine at the University of California at San Francisco, senior scientist at the Natural Resources Defense Council in San Francisco, and coauthor of *Generations at Risk: Reproductive Health and the Environment.*

"Some scientists squint at this half-completed puzzle and see a pattern," she says. "Others squint at the same assortment of pieces and say, 'It's a random mess; I don't see anything.' Right now, many scientists, myself included, are

WOMEN ASK WHY

How can I find out what chemicals are used in my community?

Unless you live in Massachusetts or Oregon—the two states that require chemical reporting—you'll have a hard time finding out what chemicals are used in your area. Those states require larger companies to report any toxic chemical *use*, but most states require companies to report only toxic chemicals they *release*. In other words, in the other 48 states, companies have to report only what comes out of their plants in the smoke and water and onto the land.

However, you should have the *right* to know what harmful chemicals you're being exposed to. Many people are endangered by toxic chemicals in their jobs. Others are imperiled by using inadequately labeled products. This is not right. In medicine, for example, it is unethical to treat people with drugs or to experiment on them without their complete consent. Yet this same society allows its citizens to be regularly exposed in other facets of their lives to dangerous and inadequately tested substances without being told and without their consent.

So what can you do? Sadly, there's no one source for information on toxic hazards. A good place to start, however, is the Environmental Protection Agency (EPA). Write to 401 M Street, S.W., Washington, DC 20460. Or check out the

putting those pieces together. We're looking at the increasing rates of birth defects of the reproductive tract in humans and the similar findings in lab animals and wildlife exposed to endocrine disrupters. And we're saying, 'There's a pattern.'

"We're not saying that we have absolute scientific proof from what we know so far," she continues. "But we are saying that there's enough information to take some prudent action."

One thing researchers do know: The developing fetus—animal or human—is most vulner-

Web site at www.epa.gov. It contains a link called Your Community. Type in your zip code for a list of facilities in your area regulated by the EPA and for such information as whether or not any toxic releases have been reported from the facilities.

Another good source is the Agency for Toxic Substances and Disease Registry (ATSDR), U.S. Department of Health and Human Services, 1600 Clifton Road, N.E., Atlanta, GA 30333; (888) 42-ATSDR. This agency conducts public health assessments of waste sites and provides fact sheets on more than 100 toxic chemicals. Or visit the Web site at www.atsdr.cdc.gov. Click on Resources to view the Hazardous Substance Release and Health Effects Database.

It's easier to find out what's in your drinking water. The EPA requires that water suppliers send their customers an annual water quality report. This report discloses chemicals and contaminants in your water. Contact your water supplier to get a copy or check for it online at www.epa.gov. If your water isn't safe to drink, your water supplier is required to notify you by newspaper, mail, radio, TV, or hand delivery.

Expert consulted
Ted Schettler, M.D.
Science director
Science and Environmental Health Network
Coauthor of Generations at Risk: Reproductive Health and the Environment

United States in 1977. It's thought they interfere with thyroid hormone function during critical periods of fetal brain development.

Hormonal Havoc at Home?

One reason we still don't know whether low concentrations of many HAAs have health effects is that, despite some studies, experts still don't have a complete picture of what our overall exposure actually *is*, and we don't comprehensively track health effects that might be caused by low-level exposures.

In an attempt to learn whether synthetic chemicals might behave as HAAs, the Environmental Protection Agency (EPA) formed a panel of experts, the Endocrine Disrupter Screening and Testing Advisory Committee, to recommend a screening and testing program for thousands of chemicals. Of particular concern are pesticides used on food and common contaminants of drinking water. The committee presented its recommendations to the EPA in 1999. Although the EPA is standardizing and validating the recommended tests, a comprehensive screening program is still years away.

Other EPA studies suggest that levels of indoor air pollutants may be 25 times—and occasionally more than 100 times—higher than outdoor levels. Not a pleasant thought given that most of us spend up to 90 percent of our time indoors.

While we may be most concerned about these chemicals' effects on our own and our family's health, we should also consider their impact on

able to HAAs. Researchers who study HAAs identify windows of vulnerability during which these chemicals can damage a fetus's intellectual development, its endocrine or immune system, or its later ability to reproduce.

For instance, children born to Michigan women who had high levels of the HAA polychlorinated biphenyls (PCBs) in their blood—mostly from eating fish from the Great Lakes—have IQs an average of 6 points lower than children whose mothers had lower PCB levels. PCBs were banned from most uses in the

others in our communities and on local animals, fish, and wildlife, says Dr. Solomon.

"We can't protect ourselves and our families by walling ourselves off," she says. "We have to think as a community and try to make changes that will help everybody." Sounds like activism? It is—of a sort, says Dr. Solomon. "Activism doesn't have to mean hitting the streets. Something as simple as attending a PTA meeting and trying to get your child's school to stop using pesticides on its playground can help everyone in your community."

There's no way to rid our homes of *every* potentially toxic chemical, HAA or otherwise, unless we'd be willing to trade in our houses for plastic bubbles. But we *can* identify known or suspected HAAs and take steps to avoid them, says Dr. Solomon. It's what scientists call the "precautionary principle" and what we might term the "better-safe-than-sorry" principle. Let's take a room-by-room environmental tour of a typical home—perhaps your home—for ideas.

Your Kitchen

Here's an irony for you. The kitchen, where you prepare your healthy meals, contains a number of HAAs.

Pesticides on fruits and vegetables. Remember DDT? The EPA does. The agency banned use of this pesticide in 1972 because it was decimating wildlife ecology, especially bird populations. Unfortunately, DDT tends to stick around, both in the environment and in our bodies, where it's stored in fat and tissue. In fact, in 1997, DDT was found in 24 percent of 1,036 food samples tested by the FDA for pesticides and other chemical residues.

What's more, several pesticides now in use have also been shown to be HAAs. Methoxychlor and endosulfan are estrogenic, while atrazine, simazine, and cyanazine alter the metabolism of estrogen and testosterone. Prelimi-

nary studies on the effects of pesticides in people have found a link between exposure to these pesticides and breast and ovarian cancers.

To remove pesticide residues from fruits and vegetables:

→ Rinse, don't soak. Running water acts as an abrasive, helping to remove residue.

→ Peel your produce.

→ Eat a wide range of fruits and vegetables. Because specific pesticides are used for specific crops, a varied diet can prevent you from consuming too much of any one pesticide.

→ Buy organically grown food—plant foods grown and processed without the use of synthetic fertilizers or pesticides. For more on organic food, see Safeguard Your Diet against Hormones on page 155.

→ Eat fewer apples, apricots, bell peppers (from the United States and Mexico), cantaloupes (from Mexico), celery, cherries (from the United States), cucumbers, grapes (from Chile), green beans, peaches, spinach, and strawberries. Based on FDA and EPA data, the Environmental Working Group in Washington, D.C., found that these fruits and vegetables consistently contain the most pesticide residues.

Bisphenol A. It's found in items such as plastic food storage containers, food and drink containers, the linings of food and drink cans, and clear baby bottles. Bisphenol A is a potent estrogen, says Frederick S. vom Saal, Ph.D., professor of biology at the University of Missouri in Columbia, who has been studying the effects of this chemical.

Dr. vom Saal and his colleagues, along with researchers at North Carolina State University, exposed pregnant mice to the same levels of bisphenol A that we typically encounter. They found that the chemical caused the mice offspring to grow faster after birth and to enter puberty earlier than normal.

Exposure to bisphenol A may be one reason girls in the United States are entering puberty at a younger age, says Dr. vom Saal. Further, the chemical may increase our risk of breast cancer, by increasing our lifetime exposure to estrogen.

Di (ethylhexyl) adipate (DEHA). Some household and commercial cling wraps—such as the plastic film supermarkets use to wrap cheeses and meats—are made of polyvinyl chloride (PVC) that contains the plasticizer DEHA, a chemical that lubricates the wrap and makes it more pliable. Animal studies suggest that DEHA is another type of endocrine disrupter. Other research has shown that DEHA can leach into food wrapped in plastic.

To use plastics safely:

- Use plastic wraps made of polyethylene, which don't contain plasticizers. Check the product's packaging for a customer service number and direct questions on content to the individual company.
- Don't allow the plastic wrap to touch the food when microwaving.
- Immediately remove cling wrap from deli meats and cheeses and transfer them to aluminum foil or wax paper.
- Use a cheese slicer to shave off a layer of the surface of hard cheeses wrapped in plastic. This can remove DEHA.
- Microwave only in containers labeled as safe for use in the appliance.
- Don't reuse the plastic trays that come with frozen microwave dinners.
- Don't microwave food in margarine tubs or dairy containers (such as yogurt containers). They aren't heat tested and could allow chemicals to leach into food.

Your Bathroom

In the 1980s, the EPA conducted a series of studies—called the Total Exposure Assessment Methodology—to measure people's total exposure to two dozen common volatile organic compounds (VOCs), including chloroform. These compounds are volatile by definition and may have toxic properties. However, very little is known about the possible hormone-disrupting effects of many VOCs. That's why the screening and testing program is necessary.

The researchers found chloroform—a by-product of water chlorination—in all the tap water tested. They also found that the total dose of chloroform (along with other VOCs) a woman receives from showering with contaminated water is roughly equal to that of drinking two liters of the water.

Nobody's saying to stop showering. But this little statistic serves to illustrate just how environmentally ubiquitous VOCs are. (And don't panic; there are ways to de-chloroform your baths and showers, too.)

Other toxins, including potential HAAs, in your john include:

Phthalates. They're in nail polish, hair spray, hand lotion, and perfume. There's virtually no research on the human health effects of these chemicals—also widely used in household products, clothing, toys, and other products. But in animal studies, exposure to even small amounts of some of these substances caused defects in male offspring.

Further, a recent government review of phthalates concluded that at least a few of these substances—notably di-2-ethylhexyl phthalate (DEHP)—have the potential to cause birth defects or reproductive problems in human male fetuses.

Apparently, we receive more exposure to more types of phthalates than experts previously knew. Using a new technique, researchers for the Centers for Disease Control (CDC) were able to measure the presence of metabolites, or the breakdown products, of seven types of phthalates in human urine.

The phthalates found at the highest levels, diethyl phthalate (DEP) and dibutyl phthalate (DBP), are used extensively in perfumes, soaps, nail polish, and hair sprays.

What's more, women of childbearing age were found to have the highest urinary levels of monobutyl phthalate, a breakdown product of DBP and a reproductive and developmental toxin in animals.

Should we give up manicures, hair spray, and perfume? There's no clear-cut answer.

"This is an exposure study. It doesn't tell us anything about phthalates' health effects," says study coauthor John Brock, Ph.D., senior chemist and team leader of the phthalates project for the CDC in Chamblee, Georgia. "When we have incomplete information, such as with phthalates, we have to make our own decisions," says Dr. Brock.

Alkylphenol exthoxylates (APEs). You'll find them in air fresheners, toilet-bowl deodorizers, and surface disinfectants. These chemicals—used widely in a variety of cleaning and personal care products, including hair coloring and hair conditioners—are surfactants, which means they help oil and water mix.

Some APEs, such as octyl phenol and nonylphenol, are estrogenic. While there has been no research on their effects in humans, exposure to these compounds reduces the size of testicles in male fish and rats and the daily sperm production in male rats. In another study, nonylphenol caused estrogen-sensitive cells to grow in both test tubes and in the uteruses of rats, which could theoretically increase cancer risk.

"There's no direct evidence that APEs affect our hormonal health," says Dr. Solomon. "But what's bad for fish and rats may ultimately turn out to be not very good for people."

To "de-HAA" your bathroom:
- Buy filters for your shower and taps to keep out chlorine. Carbon filters remove some

VOCs, including chloroform. Solid-block and precoat-activated carbon filters also reduce heavy metals such as lead and mercury. (Not all carbon filtration systems capture heavy metals or minerals.) If you don't have a water filter and your water is chlorinated, run the bathroom exhaust fan as you shower. Enclosed areas concentrate the chloroform more than open ones. And if you're relaxing in a bath, open the window. Weather permitting, you should be doing this anyway to help reduce moisture and mold.

- Color your nails naturally with a henna nail paste, suggests Greta Breedlove, in her book *The Herbal Home Spa: Naturally Refreshing Wraps, Rubs, Lotions, Masks, Oils, and Scrubs.* Place 1 tablespoon of henna (available at health food and cosmetics stores) in a small dish and add 1 tablespoon of water. Then add 2 drops of vitamin E oil to form a paste. Using a small brush, paint the paste onto your nails. (Wash off any spills as soon as they occur; henna stains skin.) Allow the henna to dry at least 20 minutes, then buff your nails with a nail buffer.

- Buy environmentally friendly cleaners. Two companies that offer them are Seventh Generation (www.seventhgen.com) and The Green Mercantile (www.greenmercantile.com). You can buy their products online or look for them in natural food and grocery stores nationwide.

- Make your own natural disinfectant. Add ½ teaspoon of tea tree oil (available in health food stores) to 1 gallon of distilled white vinegar, suggests Karen Logan in her book *Clean House, Clean Planet: Clean Your House for Pennies a Day the Safe, Nontoxic Way.* Tea tree oil has antiseptic properties and effectively fights both bacterial and fungal infections. You can use the disinfectant on floors, tubs, anywhere. If there's any left over, pour it into a squirt bottle for next time.

- Make a natural toilet-bowl cleaner by pouring ½ cup of borax (found in the laundry section of supermarkets) directly into your toilet. Add 20 to 30 drops of tea tree oil and swish.

Your Family Room

If your kitchen isn't the epicenter of your home, your family room probably is. It's where you and your family read, eat, watch TV, hang out.

And like the other rooms in your home, it most likely contains HAAs. Rugs are a major contributor. Dusty rugs trap pesticides and PCBs, and the thicker the pile, the more of these chemicals they're likely to harbor. This is particularly worrisome if you have an infant or toddler—or a grandchild—who crawls and plays on the rug, ingesting and breathing in the dust.

New carpets aren't much better. For a few weeks after installation, most carpets are thought to emit low amounts of VOCs, including formaldehyde from the glue used in the rugs' backing. "Another chemical, perfluoroctane sulfonate, used in some of 3M Company's Scotchgard stain-repellent products, was found to linger in human body fat over time. The company voluntarily

WOMAN TO WOMAN

She Learned to Avoid Environmental Irritants

Sharon, 50, of northeast Pennsylvania, has always reacted badly to strong scents and fragrances. As a kid, she got queasy from the odor of crayons. Today, liquid-marking pens, photocopier fumes, and perfume worn by co-workers make her light-headed and irritate her airways. A serious bout with bronchial asthma at age 47 left her airways hypersensitive and her lungs chronically inflamed. Any encounter with a strong odor—even if it's natural—triggers nonstop coughing fits. Here's how she copes.

There's really no medication for my problem. I've tried inhalers—bronchodilating medicine prescribed for asthma—but the propellants make my coughing worse, not better. My only recourse is avoiding triggers and "immunizing" myself with herbs and nutritional supplements.

After dealing with hyperactive airways for so long, I pretty much know what to avoid. Going to smoky bars or restaurants is out of the question, of course. I have to skip church on Easter Sunday—the banks of lilies in the sanctuary trigger symptoms. I buy unscented cosmetics, shampoos, and laundry detergent. I use unscented candles. In supermarkets, I try to get through the aisle with laundry detergents and cleaning products as quickly as possible. At home, we haven't used our fireplace for 2 or 3 years. Taking a job in a large city would be out of the question because of car exhaust and other air pollutants.

To help fight inflammation, I take vitamin C with quercetin, a flavonoid derived from food that acts as a natural anti-inflammatory. I also take flaxseed oil capsules, which fight inflammation, and lobelia, an herb known for relieving respiratory problems.

I'm at my best when I'm away from buildings and civilization and out in fresh air—sailing, for example, or skiing in the mountains. But until my doctor writes a prescription for me to move to the Rockies, I have to make the best of it and try to avoid putting myself in situations I know aren't good for me.

stopped manufacturing those items at the end of 2000," says Dr. Solomon.

Finally, pressed-wood furniture and paneling can also emit formaldehyde and other VOCs.

To minimize exposure to HAAs in your family room or living room:

➧ Remove your shoes before you enter your house. One study found that dust vacuumed from a living-room carpet contained 16 types of pesticides, some of which had been banned for years. Another study showed that removing shoes can reduce lead levels in carpets by 90 percent.

➧ Make your next carpet wool, if you can afford it. "Wool carpets are not treated with stain repellents. The natural lanolin in the wool is as effective as a synthetic stain repellent," says Dr. Solomon. "Nylon carpets are sprayed with stain repellents." If you can't afford wool, consider purchasing a wool-nylon blend. "Many of them are also not treated because of their wool content," says Dr. Solomon.

➧ Ask that a new carpet be unrolled and aired out before it's installed. And if glues or adhesives are needed to install it, ask that non-formaldehyde or water-based varieties be used.

➧ During and after carpet installation, open your windows and use fans to move fumes outdoors. Keep them running for 2 or 3 days after the new carpet is installed. Air conditioners with fan settings can also be used.

➧ Reconsider buying products made of pressed wood, such as furniture, cabinetry, or building materials. If you're in the market

---

HORMONES THROUGH HISTORY
DES

DES (diethylstilbestrol) was the first synthetic estrogen. It was prescribed for more than 30 years to an estimated 8 million pregnant women in the United States to help them avoid miscarriages. In 1971, it was found to be not only ineffective but also dangerous. And it was dangerous not only to the women who took it, according to later research, but also to their babies—and perhaps even to their grandchildren.

DES was first given in 1938 to women with a history of problem miscarriages, under the assumption that the supplemental estrogen would ward off miscarriages caused by hormonal imbalances. Soon, because it was considered safe and effective, doctors also began prescribing it for healthy mothers. Suddenly, pharmacists couldn't fill DES prescriptions fast enough.

As the wave of prescriptions continued to increase in the 1950s, however, so did the questions surrounding the drug's efficacy. Then a landmark study at the University of Chicago compared 840 pregnant women given DES with 806 pregnant women given a placebo (inactive substitute). Results proved DES didn't prevent premature births or miscarriages. Subsequent studies confirmed the drug's ineffectiveness,

---

for a new entertainment center or computer table, check the Web for manufacturers of environmentally friendly furniture. Or simply buy new or used furniture made of solid wood.

Your Bedroom

Poke your head into your closet. If you're overpowered by the odor of freshly dry-cleaned clothing, you're getting a whiff of a probable carcinogen and a suspected HAA. In recent years, the chemical the majority of dry cleaners use—perchloroethylene (PCE)—has come under gov-

but DES continued to be prescribed until 1971. Only when the Food and Drug Administration found a link between DES and a rare form of vaginal cancer, clear cell adenocarcinoma (CCAC), in the daughters of the women who took DES did it ban the drug's use in pregnant women. At that time, 21 cases of CCAC in DES-exposed daughters had been reported. Ten years later, more than 400 cases had been found, as well as other reproductive abnormalities, miscarriages, and premature births in those daughters. Additionally, National Cancer Institute researchers found that DES mothers had a 20 to 30 percent increased risk of breast cancer as they aged.

But the questions continue. In 1999, participants at the DES Research Update Conference held at the National Institutes of Health in Bethesda, Maryland, agreed to examine the grandchildren of DES moms to see if they had an increased risk of testicular cancer or other reproductive problems and autoimmune diseases. Conference researchers also agreed they need to determine whether other compounds such as drugs, pesticides, or other agents may have DES-like adverse effects. Because many Americans aren't aware of DES and its effects, the health research community is developing national education programs. If you'd like to know more about DES, go to www.desaction.org or call (800) DES-9288.

To reduce your risk of exposure:

- Before you wear freshly dry-cleaned clothing or put it into your closet, air it out—preferably outdoors.
- If your clothing has a strong chemical odor when you pick it up from the dry cleaner, don't take it. Ask that they keep it for a couple of days and air it out—and educate them on the hazards of PCE exposure.
- If you live near a dry cleaner, call an indoor-air testing company and have your home tested for PCE contamination, especially if you're pregnant, trying to become pregnant, or breastfeeding.
- Search for a dry cleaner who uses liquid carbon dioxide, the same stuff used to carbonate sodas, or "wet cleaning" technologies. One such chain, Hangers Cleaners, can be found online at www.hangers-drycleaners.com.

Your Laundry Room

Chances are you've got APEs lurking in your laundry room in the form of detergents and spot removers.

"Since APEs are surfactants, they help water mix into and lift out dirt and stains," says Dr. Solomon.

ernment scrutiny and regulation as scientific research reveals evidence of its risks to our health and environment. In 1996, almost 8 million pounds of PCE were released into the air, land, and water. This chemical accumulates in our bodies and has been found in blood, tissue, exhaled breath, and breast milk. Studies of dry-cleaning workers have connected PCE exposure to a variety of serious health problems, from headaches and nausea to an increased risk of several types of cancer.

There's also strong evidence that exposure to PCE may increase the risk of infertility (in both women and men) and miscarriage.

Manufacturers aren't required to list APEs on the label. But if you don't want them in your detergents, call your brand's consumer help line and ask if the product contains APEs, says Philip Dickey, Ph.D., of the Washington Toxics Coalition in Seattle and author of the report *Troubling Bubbles: The Case for Replacing Alkylphenol Ethoxylate (APE) Surfactants.*

If your brand does contain the chemical, let

the manufacturer know you're concerned. "These calls can help manufacturers understand that consumers would rather not have these chemicals in their products," says Dr. Dickey.

To drive APEs out of your laundry room:

- Use less detergent. According to environmentalists, the amount recommended on the label is usually twice what you need to wash an average load.
- Make an all-natural laundry soap. Blend 1 cup of soap flakes (available in the supermarket) with 1 cup of baking soda and 1 cup of washing soda (sodium carbonate, also known as sal soda). This should make enough for six average wash loads, using ½ cup of the mixture per load. Store in a heavy plastic container. To scent your suds, blend 3 to 5 drops of an essential oil such as Texas or Virginian cedarwood (adds a clean, woodsy scent), tea tree (an antibacterial), or lavender (just because it smells good) with the above mixture.
- Consider using white vinegar as a natural fabric softener. To give it a fresh scent, mix 20 drops of lavender essential oil into 1 gallon of white vinegar. For a large load, use 1 cup during the rinse cycle; smaller loads, ½ cup.

Your Lawn and Garden

We all want prizewinning tomatoes and lush, weed-free lawns. To get them, however, we spent over a billion dollars in 1993 for 71 million pounds of pesticides, much of which ended up on our yards.

We've already discussed the potential health risks of pesticides. So you may want to consider a method that can give pests the boot without resorting to chemical warfare: integrated pest management (IPM), which focuses on preventing pest damage before it starts. According to the EPA, it's the most effective pest-control method there is.

To incorporate IPM techniques into your lawn and garden care:

- Select healthy seeds that are known to resist diseases and are suited to your climate. They're likely to produce strong, hardy plants that don't need pesticides.
- If you have a large garden, alternate rows of different kinds of plants. Pests that prefer tomatoes, for instance, may not get all of them if other veggies are planted in neighboring rows.
- Choose a type of grass that grows well in your climate. Your local county cooperative extension service can tell you which varieties grow best in your area.
- Grow your grass a bit longer. That makes it harder for weeds to take root and grow. Aim for 2½ to 3½ inches long before cutting.

If you must use pesticides:

- Never apply pesticides on a windy day. Position yourself so that even a light breeze doesn't blow the spray or dust into your face.
- If spraying a pesticide, use a coarse-droplet nozzle on your sprayer. This helps keep you from inhaling mist.
- Never mix or apply a pesticide near a well.
- When you're done, rinse tools and equipment in a bucket *three times*. Rinse the containers and utensils you used to mix the pesticide, too.
- Wash your hands after applying any pesticide. And take off your shoes or boots before going inside so you don't track pesticides indoors.
- If you have leftover pesticide, follow the label's disposal directions. If you don't have the original container, call your local environmental agency or health department for help.

Safeguard Your Diet against Hormones

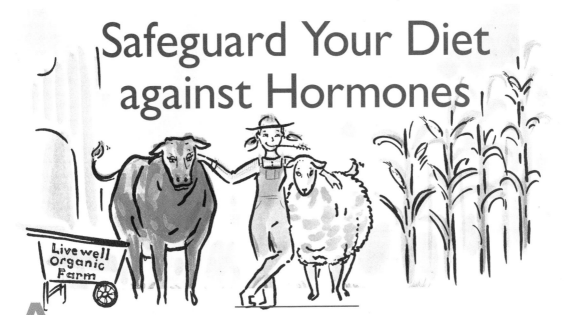

Live well Organic Farm

As women, we take pride in cooking healthy meals for our families. From fruits and veggies to grains, meat, and dairy, we want them to get the vitamins and minerals they need to stay strong and well.

But have you ever wondered if you're getting more than you planned in your family dinners? Just what *is* in regular milk and meat that makes their organic counterparts so strongly emphasize "no antibiotics, no hormones" on their packages?

"People are of the opinion that no risk is acceptable when it comes to food," says Tim Zacharewski, Ph.D., an associate professor in the department of biochemistry and molecular biology at Michigan State University in East Lansing and an expert on chemicals that affect our hormones. "What they don't realize is that there are risks associated with all foods, including organic fruits and vegetables. The idea that organic fruits and vegetables are healthier or safer and that genetically modified foods are unsafe is extremely exaggerated."

Here's what we do know: Despite all the headlines, food in the United States is very safe, thanks to federal protections.

Everything else, it seems, depends on whom you talk to. But regardless, there are things you can look for and do to ensure that you and your family eat not only the very safest of the safe but also the very tastiest of the tasty when you sit down to a meal.

Hormonal Influences

It's one thing to get Cajun seasoning with that chicken. It's quite another to get hormones. Just seeing the word used in the same sentence as any type of food brings worries about its effect on our health, including increased risks of cancer and reproductive problems.

Some may be well-founded.

In 1979, the U.S. Department of Health and Human Services told farmers they could no longer give beef cattle or any other food-producing animal a hormone called diethylstilbestrol (DES) to promote growth. Why? When given to pregnant women to prevent miscarriages and other complications, this potent man-made estrogen increased their chances of getting breast cancer by 30 percent. It also put their un-

WOMAN TO WOMAN

Going Vegan Ended Her Endometriosis

For years, Joi Straaten, now 35, dreaded getting her period. Her severe endometriosis (a gynecological condition in which tissue that's usually inside the uterus grows outside the uterine cavity) left her in such excruciating pain that she couldn't leave her bed several days a month. Even worse, it was preventing her from getting pregnant, despite years of trying. At the end of her rope, Joi went one step beyond her vegetarianism and became a vegan—someone who eats no animal or dairy products. Within a few months, her periods became regular and pain-free, and today, the Sandy, Utah, resident is the mom of two healthy daughters. Here is her story.

When I decided to go vegan, I had been trying to get pregnant for about 10 years. Three doctors had told me I would not be able to have children. One suggested I have a hysterectomy when I was 25 because my endometriosis was so bad. But I kept on trying, undergoing surgery for the endometriosis in 1992 and 1995. After the operation, my doctor advised 6 months of hormone shots to keep the endometriosis from returning.

The shots were awful. They basically brought on menopause—hot flashes, night sweats, erratic periods. After 4 months, I couldn't deal with the side effects any longer, and I bought *Women's Bodies, Women's Wisdom: Creating Physical and Emotional Health and Healing* by Christiane Northrup, M.D. The first thing she recommends for endometriosis? Eliminate dairy and see what happens. So I did, buying soy milk, tofu cheese, soy yogurt, and soy ice cream instead.

When I returned to my doctor for my fourth hormone shot, I told him I didn't want any more injections. He was furious and warned me the endometriosis would come back even worse. But I was convinced eating vegan was worth a try.

I was right. Six months later, my doctor—much to his shock—found no signs of the endometriosis. One year later, he told me there was no reason why I couldn't get pregnant—this from the man who'd told my husband and me to start pursuing adoption.

Within 2 weeks, I conceived.

Fifteen months after Ruby was born, I got pregnant again. Lilah Rose was born in August 1999.

born sons and daughters at risk for reproductive cancers and abnormalities. These findings concerned regulators, who suspected that DES might also be powerful enough to harm the unborn baby of a woman who ate DES-treated beef.

Our beef cattle don't receive DES anymore (and neither do pregnant women), but cows do get other estrogenic ("female") and androgenic ("male") hormones before they end up on our dinner tables. They start receiving these hormones—generally through implants in their ears—when they're about 6 months old. These drugs, some natural and some synthetic versions of the animals' own hormones, help the cattle add muscle quicker.

The practice may be spreading to the pork industry, where researchers are exploring the idea of porcine growth hormone (also known as porcine somatotropin or PST). This hormone and other substances may help pigs gain less fat and more muscle, producing leaner pork.

As disconcerting as giving hormones to food animals may sound, says Arthur L. Craigmill, Ph.D., a toxicologist at the University of California at Davis, it's a safe and closely monitored agricultural practice. "The levels are so low they're within the normal hormonal fluctuations in the animal's body," he explains. These hormones are rapidly metabolized and eliminated from the body. And if government tests do find excessive hormonal residues in an animal, its meat can't be sold for human consumption.

Just don't tell that to the Europeans. Saying that hormone-treated beef is unhealthy, the European Union has refused to accept American imports of the product. In 1999, it argued that 17-beta-estradiol, an estrogen given to U.S. beef, is a carcinogen. It believes that five other common growth hormones may also present risk.

Dr. Craigmill says the controversy is more of a trade dispute than a genuine issue. "The potential to have impact is not the same as impact," he says, noting that there are no studies supporting the Europeans' contentions.

Finally, what about chicken? Thanks to selective breeding for fast growth, "these animals have been naturally genetically engineered," says Dr. Craigmill. "They grow so fast there's no reason to put hormones in them."

A Nice Tall Glass of . . . Hormones?

Some dairy cows get their own controversial hormone treatments: recombinant bovine growth hormone (also known as recombinant bovine somatotropin) to extend the amount of milk farmers can get from older cows.

This hormone, which occurs naturally in milk, has been a source of great debate in its genetically engineered form (known as rbGH or rbST). Some fear it may increase our risk of cancer.

But others, including the FDA,

SUPER SALMON

High in healthy omega-3 fatty acids, salmon represents an increasingly popular dish on our dinner tables. At an average of $8 per pound, this fish is also one of the costliest.

That may change in the next year or two. A biotechnology company wants to bring salmon that's 40 percent cheaper to your plate. How? By adding a gene that makes the fish reach adulthood—and harvest—faster.

The process, developed by Massachusetts-based A/F Protein during the past 12 years, works like this: Scientists take a fertilized egg from an Atlantic salmon, a fish commonly farmed for food, and insert a gene that's spliced together from two different fish: the instructional part of a gene from an edible fish called the ocean pout and a growth hormone gene from a chinook salmon.

The spliced gene allows the salmon to produce growth hormone all year, instead of seasonally as the fish naturally does. As a result, these salmon become adult size in half the time it normally takes.

But don't look for these bargain fillets in the seafood case just yet—the FDA is still evaluating the product. If it's approved, though, the salmon could be the first transgenic—or genetically modified—animal food approved for human consumption.

On the health side, the FDA wants to know whether eating these fish could affect our hormones or other substances in our bodies known as growth factors.

It's understandable, especially given the debate over bovine growth hormone in milk, but the concern about hormone levels may be misplaced, says William Muir, Ph.D., a professor of genetics at Purdue University in West Lafayette, Indiana. "Any increase in growth hormones will be carefully monitored by the FDA," he says.

Instead, we should worry about the environment, Dr. Muir says. He's concerned that, if genetically modified fish escape into the wild, they could dramatically reduce wild salmon stocks if wild females were attracted to the fast-growing genetically modified male salmon.

To reduce such risks, A/F Protein plans to produce only sterile female fish.

AMERICA'S FIRST CERTIFIED ORGANIC RESTAURANT

When Nora Pouillon opened her organic restaurant in Washington, D.C., in 1979, she soon found she had some explaining to do.

"I would say, 'I have an American organic restaurant,'" Pouillon recalls. "People would say, 'Oh! I'm vegetarian, too!'"

More than 20 years later, most people now know the difference between vegetarian (no meat) and organic (produced without chemicals) food, but Pouillon is still teaching the nation's capital about eating organic. In 1999, Restaurant Nora became the country's first certified-organic restaurant.

"I wanted to bring awareness to customers that what they were eating was truly organic," Pouillon explains. "Too often, people think organic is a big hoax, that it's just a way for the farmers to get a better price." By certifying her restaurant as organic (an involved process that requires reams of paperwork and a yearly, on-site inspection), she hopes to counteract those perceptions.

But Pouillon didn't stop her education efforts at Restaurant Nora's certification stamp. Her menu, which changes daily depending on the day's deliveries, details the organic stories behind her dishes—from the free-range veal raised on mother's milk to the heirloom tomatoes grown by Amish farmers. Bottles of certified-organic olive oil sit on the white tablecloth-covered tables. Even the wine list notes those produced without chemical fertilizers or pesticides.

Developing such a diverse organic menu took time. "You can get Cheddar in a million forms, but try finding a good organic blue cheese or Camembert," Pouillon sighs. She has to order beef months in advance—and agree to buy the whole animal. "I get two filet mignons, two New York strips, two Delmonicos, and 900 pounds of ground beef," she says with a laugh.

Not surprisingly, this emphasis on quality ingredients makes for simple dishes where these foods can shine. Farm eggs cut like orange sections join a garlicky Caesar salad with wide Parmesan shavings. Slices of deep-red heirloom tomatoes mingle with fresh mozzarella and basil in a balsamic vinaigrette. After dinner, a scoop of Nora's homemade roasted banana ice cream (served atop a still-warm chocolate soufflé cake just meant for chocoholics) makes you wish for a half-gallon container and a spoon.

Add the architectural artifacts—including a weathered wooden owl overlooking the main dining room—Amish crib quilts on the walls, and the sophisticated menu (dinner entrées start in the $20 range) and you have a restaurant experience completely at odds with bare-bones organic stereotypes.

"When people see 'organic' or 'healthy' food, they think of bean sprouts and rice, Birkenstocks and macramé," says the 57-year-old Pouillon, wearing a sleek black dress and four golden rings on her hand. "I want to show them that an organic restaurant can do anything any other restaurant can do, only here they can be assured the ingredients are organic and environmentally sustainable."

say that the hormone product is not only safe when used according to label instructions but also undetectable in milk.

"You can test for rbGH/rbST," says Leslie J. Butler, Ph.D., an agricultural economist at the University of California in Davis. "It is different from naturally occurring bovine growth hormone."

Others question the hormone's safety. The European Union Scientific Committee found that milk from rbGH/rbST cows has higher levels of a natural substance known as insulin-like growth factor 1 (IGF-1). IGF-1 may be associated with higher risks of breast and gastrointestinal cancers in humans.

Often quoted, this finding remains contentious, says Dr. Butler. "The medical and scientific evidence surrounding it is tenuous," he maintains.

"The body creates its own IGF-1," Dr. Butler explains. "You don't need more unless you're diabetic." And while an excess isn't good for us, it's easily broken down by the digestive system. People with diabetes, for example, can't swallow an IGF-1 pill and expect any benefits; they must inject insulin into the bloodstream. That means drinking milk from rbGH/rbST-treated cows should be safe, Dr. Butler says, because any extra IGF-1 should get broken down in digestion before it could affect our hormones.

Yet some remain skeptical about the hormone, opting for milk that's free of rbGH/rbST until more research has been done. "If milk is not labeled rbGH/rbST-free, the only alternative for consumers is to drink organic milk," Dr. Butler says.

So far, the FDA has not required all genetically engineered foods to be labeled as such solely on the basis of being genetically engineered.

Take Control

There are things you can do about hormones in your food, experts say:

KNOW YOUR LABELS

The labels on certified-organic foods let you know just how "organic" a product is.

At its most basic, *organic* refers to food produced without man-made pesticides, herbicides, antibiotics, or hormones. But years of hopscotch state and organizational guidelines left farmers and consumers confused about just what organic really meant. So in 2000, the federal government approved national standards for certifying food as organic.

Farm animals raised for organic meat must eat organic feed and can't be given antibiotics or hormones to boost their growth. Plants must be grown without synthetic fertilizers. And genetically modified crops can't be called organic, even if they are grown using organic methods. If farmers follow all these rules, have their land free of prohibited substances for at least 3 years, and keep an extensive paper trail, they're eligible for organic certification.

That, in turn, determines how manufacturers can label their products.

Organic or 100 percent organic. Whether they're vegetables, meats, or prepared foods, they're 95 to 100 percent certified-organic ingredients, except for any water or salt.

Made with organic ingredients. These foods are 50 to 95 percent certified organic. If less than half of a food's ingredients are organic, the producer can mention them only in the ingredients list—the product can't be billed as organic.

Certified organic. Only farmers or producers who have received organic certification can use this label.

Look for "natural" or certified-organic meats. Raised without antibiotics or hormones, "natural" beef or chicken occupies the middle ground between conventionally raised and organically produced meats. If you can find organic meats, they're an even better choice because they must be raised on certified-organic feed. "Eating chicken raised in an antibiotic-free environment should reduce your personal expo-

GROWING AN ORGANIC GARDEN

Want to care for yourself emotionally as well as physically? Start an organic garden. Here's how.

Pick a sunny spot. You'll want your garden, which should be on well-drained soil (no standing water), to get 11 hours of sun daily.

Turn it over. If your garden is on what was formerly a chemically treated lawn, revitalize the soil by tilling the area, letting weeds grow, and tilling again.

Check your soil. For little or no cost, a local agricultural extension agent will test your soil's pH, providing guidance on what your garden needs to grow. "Testing now will save you heartbreak later," says Brian Cramer, production manager for vegetables and flowers at the organic Sunnyside Farms in Washington, Virginia.

Start small. A 50-square-foot plot can yield as much as 100 pounds of produce from April to October.

Think seasonal. When you grow small organic crops, you need to work with nature, not fight it with chemicals. To get the most from your garden, plant produce at appropriate times, such as lettuce in spring or arugula in fall.

Mix it up. Protect your garden from pests by planting herbs, fruits, vegetables, and flowers (such as Queen Anne's lace) in the same plot.

Let herbs bloom. Cooks often pinch herb flowers to sustain their culinary use, but Cramer recommends letting dill, cilantro, parsley, and mint plants flower—they attract beneficial insects.

Do several plantings. If insects or diseases strike your first batch of tomatoes, you'll have second and third chances to harvest your hard-earned veggies.

Cover your plants. Row covers, available in garden stores, protect young plants from harmful insects. "I religiously use them on eggplants," Cramer says.

Create compost. To enrich your soil, spread grass clippings on the garden. Or add them to a compost bin along with kitchen peelings; you can use the compost for fertilizer after 3 months. Don't compost meat scraps, though—you'll attract rodents.

sure to resistant organisms, although there's no guarantee considering the way these organisms move in nature," says Craig Hedberg, Ph.D., an associate professor of Environmental and Occupational Health at the University of Minnesota's School of Public Health in Minneapolis.

Limit your own use of antibiotics. When we feel awful, we often beg our doctors for prescriptions. By forgoing unnecessary medications when you've got a cold or the flu (which are caused by viruses anyway and hence unaffected by even the most powerful antibiotics), you can avoid contributing to antibiotic resistance.

The Glowing Soybean?

In Europe, environmental groups call genetically modified (GM) food "Frankenfood" and destroy crops. In the United States, scientists say that GM crops offer hope for feeding the world's hungry.

Meanwhile, we just want to know if GM food is safe to eat.

It's a reasonable question. More than 35 percent of the corn and almost 55 percent of the soybeans grown here are genetically modified, meaning that their DNA has been changed to make them more resistant to insects and weed killers. If you have sipped soda pop or snacked on any processed foods that contain some part of the soybean, you've probably eaten GM food.

Even some heirloom varieties of vegetables—including Golden Bantam corn and Brandywine tomatoes—qualify, since they evolved through crossbreeding and genetic exchange.

But the lightning-speed pace of the science is going beyond our everyday understanding, raising numerous questions. While we're used to growing hybrid tea roses and hybrid tomatoes, we're not used to hearing about genes being traded between plants and animals or between animals and other animals. And we don't really know how to evaluate the risks and benefits of this new technology as it goes along at a breakneck pace. "When is it okay to eat heirloom tomatoes? Modern tomatoes?" asks Peter Goldsbrough, Ph.D., a professor of horticulture at Purdue University in West Lafayette, Indiana. "When is it *not* okay to genetically modify tomatoes with a tomato gene? Another plant gene? A fish gene?"

The short answer: We're not sure, but here's how it works.

Imagine inheriting genes from your parents that made you resistant to the common cold or ensured a fast, pain-free childbirth. Talk about good genes!

That's essentially what plant scientists have done as they used genetic techniques to create corn that's resistant to insects or tomatoes that ripen more slowly so they can survive long shipping times and arrive just red enough on your grocery shelves.

Borrowing from other plants and bacteria, researchers insert the desired genes into the plant, hoping these new genes find the right spot to in-

---

FINDING ORGANIC FOOD

It's worth the effort for farmers and manufacturers to go the organic route as more and more grocery stores now stock organic products. "The demand for organics is creating the supply," says William Lockeretz, Ph.D., a professor at the School of Nutrition Science and Policy at Tufts University in Medford, Massachusetts. "Before, even if you wanted organic foods, you couldn't find them."

Today, there are numerous options for shopping organically.

Specialty supermarkets. Chains such as Whole Foods Market, Wild Oats, and Trader Joe's specialize in natural foods. Usually located in metropolitan areas, these stores sell everything that you would expect to see at the local Safeway, only with an organic label: chicken broth, produce, frozen vegetables, breakfast cereals, fresh breads, and snack foods.

Conventional grocery stores. They've started stocking organics too. Look for milk, yogurt, produce such as grapes and kiwifruit, and even frozen pizza.

Co-ops. These neighborhood markets generally offer organic foods. If you become a member, you may get small discounts on your purchases.

Farmers' markets. Small organic farms often sell direct to the consumer.

---

tegrate themselves into the plant's genetic material.

The technique is hardly foolproof; Dr. Goldsbrough describes it as "a shot in the dark." Sometimes, genes land where they have no effect. Other times, they affect the plant's growth in unintended ways.

That's especially important if you're eating a food for a specific health or nutritional benefit, such as soy for building strong bones. In one study, researchers at the Center for Ethics and Toxics in California found phytoestrogen levels in genetically modified soybeans were as much

ORGANIC LIVING

For many of us, organic food inspires an idyllic vision of agriculture and eating. "Organic farming has this mystique, like we're going back to a simpler, better era," says Abigail Salyers, Ph.D., a professor of microbiology at the University of Illinois at Urbana-Champaign.

A visit to Sunnyside Farms—425 acres of organic farmland in the shadow of Virginia's Blue Ridge Mountains—does nothing to dispel such ideas.

Peach and apple orchards cover the hillsides of Sunnyside, first established in 1720. Next to the farmhouse's stone walls, bushes of raspberries—red, purple, black, and golden—grow in thick, clustered rows. A short walk away, herbs and vegetables flourish without chemicals.

But Sunnyside's organic products include more than the expected fruits, vegetables, and herbs. The farm also produces organic eggs and beef.

Gentle brown cows graze the pastures, followed by flocks of white leghorn chickens. The chickens are accompanied by portable henhouses known as "eggmobiles" at Sunnyside and move from pasture to pasture, rejuvenating the cattle-grazed soil with their scratching and droppings even as they get fresh air and exercise.

The organic cycle continues inside the barn, where grunting pink pigs root in stalls next to the cattle, preparing straw and manure for composting and eventually for use as organic fertilizer.

Natural pesticides can be used to control weeds and insects, but organic farmers need to make sure that these products are on the approved part of the National List of Approved and Prohibited Substances (developed by the National Organics Standards Board and provided by the United States Department of Agriculture). So at Sunnyside Farms, farmers use fans and herbal products to shoo flies away from cattle.

"We believe organic farming results in a happier, healthier animal as well as a better-tasting animal," says William Cole, who owns the Washington, Virginia, farm with his family. "Besides that, it's the right thing to do."

as 20 percent lower compared with nonmodified soybeans.

That type of knowledge, while currently limited, is also crucial to women who want to *avoid* certain foods because of allergies. When agricultural researchers in the mid-1990s added a Brazil nut gene to soybeans in the hope of making the beans more nutritious, they made an unexpected—and unpleasant—discovery: People who were allergic to Brazil nuts were also allergic to the new soybeans.

Such developments concern Martha Reed Herbert, M.D., Ph.D., a pediatrician and neurology instructor at Harvard Medical School in Boston. "You could wake up feeling foggy, crummy, and tired from a low-grade food allergy and not know why," she says.

She and others also worry about the health consequences of the gene insertion process. When scientists create GM plants, they use bacteria to insert the desired genes, which are accompanied by an antibiotic marker gene that tells whether the experiment worked. These "markers" are resistant to antibiotics, which concerns physicians who are already dealing with antibiotic resistance in their patients.

"If these genes get broken down in the gut, your body might not incorporate the genes, but your intestinal bacteria might," she says. "They are very good at swapping genes."

Others say such worries are unfounded. Our digestive systems thoroughly break down any DNA we eat, whether it's genetically modified or not. Resistance genes are everywhere. So are viruses. "For example, we already eat a lot of squash with viruses on it," says Allison A. Snow, Ph.D., a professor of evolution, ecology, and organismal biology at Ohio State University in Columbus. And if genetic engineering results in fewer pesticides, we may even benefit, although others say it's too soon to know whether that will actually happen.

Many say the real question about genetically modified foods is how they will affect our earth, not our health. Despite assertions that GM plants won't get out into the environment, these crops "spread a lot more than people thought," says Dr. Snow, who worries about GM plants crossbreeding with weeds and other wild species. "That's why people are so upset in Europe. The genes are turning up before the crops have been approved."

Whether you're concerned about your health or the environment, here's what you can do:

Buy organic. Certified-organic foods, whether they're fresh or prepared, cannot contain any genetically modified ingredients.

Get vocal. Tell your elected representatives your concerns, whether it's environmental consequences or the lack of labeling for GM food you're worried about.

Hormone Discoveries of the Future

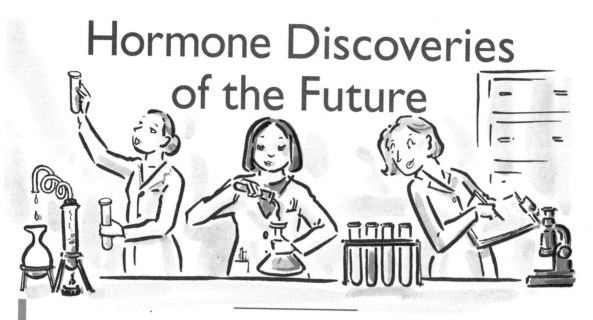

In the marathon to understand hormones and hormone-related conditions, we've only stepped up to the starting line. Many research projects have just launched, and others are but a glimmer in scientists' eyes.

But let's take a peek into the future of hormone research and see how it may affect you—from head to toe.

Gender Differences

When our brothers, husbands, or fathers do things like get up at 5:00 A.M. to play golf when it's snowing or drink the last bit of milk directly from the carton, it's easy to understand the differences between the sexes. But when it comes to pure science, researchers still can't clarify all the ways in which men and women differ.

That's because only men have been carefully studied in clinical trials. But there's pressure for this chauvinistic style of research to change. So in the future, we should have a better idea of how *women* respond to things like the latest antibiotics, heart disease medications, and even implantable devices. One specific research plan will test how all hormones—estrogens, progesterone, testosterone, prolactin, growth hormone, and insulin-like growth factor 1—react in the immune systems of both men and women.

Another gender theory to be further explored is the role of hormones in the stress response. The theory is that some hormones are responsible for men's propensity to "fight or flee," while other hormones trigger women to "tend or befriend."

"This stress theory may lead to a new understanding of some of the basic differences between men and women," says Laura Cousino Klein, Ph.D., assistant professor of behavioral health at Pennsylvania State University in University Park. She is one of six researchers who contributed to the theory.

For example, hormonal differences may explain why women want to talk out problems, while men would rather think about them alone over a beer.

"And more important, the theory may encourage researchers to further investigate the differences between men and women as they study diseases such as Alzheimer's and cancer," says Dr. Klein.

Contraception

The future of birth control also looks promising. Who knows, maybe someday people will think the condom as archaic a birth control method as the Middle Ages practice of drinking poisonous tea. Research has even progressed on a birth control pill for *men*.

"We're going to see several new delivery systems for the same kinds of hormones in oral contraceptives (estrogen and progesterone), but they'll be easier for women to use," says Susan Ballagh, M.D., of the department of obstetrics and gynecology at Eastern Virginia Medical School in Norfolk, a researcher for the Contraceptive Research and Development program funded by the U.S. Agency for International Development. Prototypes include a timed-release hormone injection, a hormone-releasing ring that's inserted into the vagina, and a birth control skin patch similar to the nicotine patch used by smokers.

More off-the-wall possibilities for the future: a soft silicone item resembling a sailor's cap that fits over the cervix, a vaginal sponge containing both a spermicide and a microbicide (so it also protects against sexually transmitted diseases), and biodegradable implants that, when inserted under the skin of the arm or hip, release progestin gradually for 12 to 18 months.

And for men? "Reversible male contraceptives would be wonderful, but whenever we do research on them, we find that anything that affects sperm also severely affects male sex drive or sexual functioning," says Marjorie Greenfield, M.D., associate professor of reproductive biology at University Hospitals of Cleveland and director of ob/gyn for DrSpock.com.

Still, research is under way at Edinburgh University to test a testosterone-containing pellet for men that's inserted into the lower abdominal wall. In one small study, 31 men received the pellet and then took oral doses of desogestrel, a new type of progestin, each day for 8 weeks. Their sperm counts fell, without negatively affecting sexual drive. Other proposals include silicone plugs to block the vas deferens tubes in the penis, through which the sperm travel, and a battery-powered capsule that emits a sperm-paralyzing electrical current when inserted into the vas deferens.

A *unisex* birth control method is also in the works. A new type of drug, called a gonadotropin releasing hormone (GnRH) agonist, prevents the release of the chemicals that trigger the production of sperm in men and ovulation in women.

Menopause

Today, menopause is just the kickoff to the *middle* of our lives, instead of signaling the end. "Women now in their fifties and sixties were raised at a time when they might have come to regard their sex organs, including the uterus, as dirty and their menses as a curse. Losing these organs as soon as they had 'done their duty' in procreation was regarded as a route to freedom from 'that mess,'" says Martha Louise Elks, M.D., professor of medicine at the Morehouse School of Medicine in Atlanta. "Now, women in their twenties and thirties find that an odd attitude."

The Study of Women's Health Across the Nation (SWAN) has set out to examine the changes we undergo during perimenopause and menopause. And there are some interesting early findings. "We classify perimenopause as a change in bleeding patterns, but we're finding that a lot of endocrinological changes are happening way before we see any bleeding changes," says Lynda

H. Powell, Ph.D., associate professor of preventive medicine at Rush–Presbyterian–St. Luke's Medical Center in Chicago, and a researcher on the study. For example, our bones may become less dense, our hormones may go haywire, and our hearts may exhibit the effects of our age way before we miss our first menstrual period. "So I think the study will ultimately change our understanding of such basic aspects of perimenopause as when it begins, its duration, and its implications," she says.

Researchers are also examining the effect of nutrition on menopause. "We need to look at what's helpful in societies where women have less-pronounced menopause symptoms and ill health and then figure out the components of the foods that cause the effects," says Ellen W. Seely, M.D., director of clinical research in the endocrine-hypertension division at Brigham and Women's Hospital in Boston.

Diabetes

When it comes to type 2 diabetes, we've come a long way, but in the wrong direction—*more* of us now get it.

"It's unbelievable now that we have 17- and 18-year-olds who have type 2, or adult-onset, diabetes. This never used to happen until people were in their forties or fifties," says Ann Zerr, M.D., clinical director of the National Center of Excellence in Women's Health at Indiana University School of Medicine in Indianapolis. A primary cause of type 2 diabetes is obesity—fueled by super-sized fast food meals and

VIAGRA AND OTHER SEX DRUGS FOR WOMEN

When Viagra came on the scene, you would've thought the drug company, Pfizer, had reinvented sex. Men reclaimed their erections proudly, and the little blue pill was hailed as the savior of marriages.

But aren't we forgetting someone in that equation?

"Research on women's sexuality lags 20 years behind that for men, even though sexual dysfunction is 30 percent more common in women than in men," says Barbara Bartlik, M.D., assistant professor of psychiatry at the Weill Medical College of Cornell University in New York City.

Thankfully, changes are afoot. Drug companies have caught on to the fact that a huge untapped market exists—some estimates say 10 million women between 50 and 75 with sexual dysfunction are clamoring for treatments. Some currently under development for women include:

Viagra. It's a vasodilator, meaning it dilates blood vessels, improving blood flow. Because Viagra's main action takes place "down south," it increases lubrication and sensation—and for some women, even their ability to reach orgasm, says Laura Berman, Ph.D., co-director of the Women's Sexual Health Clinic at the Boston University Medical Center. Dr. Berman says the best candidate for Viagra is a woman who was satisfied with her sex life in the past but who isn't able to respond as she once did—whether it's due to hysterectomy, menopause, pelvic surgery, or injury.

Although Viagra is not currently approved for use in women, many clinical trials are under way, Dr. Berman says. Still, some doctors have already begun prescribing it for women.

Testosterone. "According to current guidelines, Estratest, which contains conjugated estrogen and methyltestosterone, should be prescribed only for women who have vaginal symptoms that are not responding to estrogen replacement, but that's a joke," says Dr. Bartlik. "Ninety percent of women taking Estratest are doing it for their libidos."

But more research is still needed. We know that women who get too much testosterone experience hair growth, clitoral enlargement, and growth of the larynx, which may cause the voice to deepen. No connection has been made to heart disease or cancer in women, but women with these risk factors should be monitored closely or avoid this treatment altogether, says Dr. Bartlik.

Because oral testosterone has to pass through your digestive system, it may not be as effective as topical—plus, it could cause damage to your liver, where it is metabolized. Dr. Bartlik prescribes a testosterone gel or cream for her female patients, who apply it directly to their clitoris and vagina or inner thigh.

Prostaglandin E-1. This naturally occurring vasodilator is normally used as a suppository or injection for men to increase penile blood flow. But some doctors are enthusiastic about prostaglandin E-1's effect when applied to women's genitals, says Dr. Bartlik. Some pharmaceutical companies are working on creams and gels for women.

Apomorphine. This drug, originally developed for people with Parkinson's disease, works by encouraging release of dopamine, a pleasure-seeking neurotransmitter that can boost sexual drive and excitement and make orgasms easier to achieve. While it has not been tested in women for sexual function, it has been tested in men, with positive results. Some doctors think it may be useful in women, either alone or in combination with Viagra-like drugs.

Bupropion. This antidepressant also works by stimulating release of dopamine, but unlike its Prozac-like antidepressant colleagues, it does not negatively impact libido—in fact, it may enhance it. Bupropion is sold as an antidepressant under the name Wellbutrin and as a smoking cessation aid under the name Zyban. Some doctors prescribe it specifically for sexual dysfunction.

Phentolamine. This drug, which causes smooth muscles like those in the vagina to relax, was shown in a pilot study to increase vaginal blood flow and arousal in menopausal women with sexual dysfunction. Plans to develop a vaginal suppository form are being discussed.

hours in front of the DVD player. We don't know if restaurant portions will continue to expand in the future, but we do know that a large part of diabetes research will focus on how to shrink our society down to a healthy size.

The most important effort is to prevent type 2 diabetes, with emphasis on lifestyle changes. Other research will address ways to avoid complications once the disease shows up, says Lynne M. Kirk, M.D., associate chief of the division of internal medicine at the University of Texas Southwestern Medical Center in Dallas.

Doctors are also exploring the possible genetic causes of type 2 diabetes, such as how our own insulin works in our bodies and how we can keep ourselves from becoming insulin resistant, a leading risk factor for type 2 diabetes. "There's a lot of research into how to increase insulin production in the body," says James Rosenzweig, M.D., senior physician at the Joslin Diabetes Center in Boston. Transplantation of insulin-producing islet cells is currently in the works. When that is achieved, a further advance will be to culture islet cells outside the body to make them insulin sensitive before reintroducing them to the pancreas.

Heart Disease

Heart disease is the number one cause of death in women. Thankfully, with organizations like WomenHeart and studies like the Women's Health Initiative (WHI), our hearts are starting to receive slightly more attention.

The Women's Health Initiative, sponsored by the National Institutes of Health in Bethesda, Maryland, is studying 161,000 women ages 50 to 79 to, among other things, better understand estrogen's effect on the heart. Early results suggest that estrogen may not be as protective as once thought.

"But one of the big issues with estrogen is that maybe you don't see protection in the first 3 years (the length of the study as of 2000), but you see it in 10 years," says Dr. Seely.

It may also be the way postmenopausal women take hormone replacement therapy that's associated with a lack of protection. "We give people pills to take that have very little to do with what their bodies were doing premenopausally," says Dr. Seely. "So maybe if we gave postmenopausal women hormones more like the naturally occurring estradiol and progesterone that their bodies made when they were younger, the hormones would provide better protection against heart disease."

Mood Disorders

Researchers have begun to examine the link between oxytocin, the hormone we produce during labor and lactation, and mood disorders such as depression. This could help explain the cause of postpartum depression, for example.

And at the University of California at San Francisco, Owen M. Wolkowitz, M.D., a professor of psychiatry, is looking at stress hormones like cortisol and DHEA and their roles in depression. These studies and similar ones by other researchers will likely lead to new treatments, including new prescription drugs for depression, anxiety, and other mood disorders, he says.

Cancer

In the arena of cancer and hormones, there are numerous stones yet to be overturned. The Women's Insights and Shared Experiences study at the University of Pennsylvania, designed to determine the role of hormones and genes in breast and endometrial cancers, may lead to a greater understanding of why we get cancer in the first place. This, in turn, could lead to better cancer-prevention drugs. Other studies are also under way to investigate the role of estrogen in colon and lung cancers.

Osteoporosis

Research is under way to discover better ways to keep our bones healthy, test bone quality, and treat the bones when they begin to thin. In just the past decade, enormous strides have been realized, including drugs to stop bones from deteriorating, but there are none that actually rebuild bone.

"I expect they will find something to build bone in the next 5 years," Manish Suthar, M.D., physician at the Texas Back Institute in Plano, said in late 2000. "There are a variety of agents being studied that actually build bone. One example is fluoride."

In the osteoporosis prevention arena, there's magnesium. Along with calcium, it can help prevent the disease. "I think in the near future, more people will take magnesium to prevent osteoporosis," says Maria Sulindro, M.D., president and founder of eAntiAging.com, an Internet organization that provides scientific information about antiaging approaches.

Safe Use of Herbs

While herbs are generally safe and cause few, if any, side effects, researchers and specialists in natural medicine caution that you should use them responsibly. Foremost, if you are under a doctor's care for any health condition or are on any medication, don't take any herb without telling your doctor. Certain natural substances can change the way your body absorbs and processes some medications. Also, if you are pregnant, don't self-treat with any natural remedy without the consent of your obstetrician or midwife. The same goes if you are nursing or attempting to conceive.

Every product has the potential to cause adverse reactions. Below are cautions for herbs mentioned in this book that may be more likely than others to cause adverse reactions in some people. (The list covers only those herbs and is not comprehensive.) Though such occurrences are rare, you should be aware that they exist and discontinue use of the herb if you experience an unusual reaction. Also, don't exceed the recommended dosages—more is *not* better. By familiarizing yourself with this list, you can enjoy the world of natural healing and use this book with confidence.

Herb	Safety Guidelines and Possible Side Effects
American ginseng (*Panax quinquefolium*)	May cause irritability if taken with caffeine or other stimulants. Do not take if you have high blood pressure.
Asian or Korean ginseng (*Panax ginseng*)	May cause irritability if taken with caffeine or other stimulants. Do not take if you have high blood pressure.
Black cohosh (*Actea racemosa*)	Do not use for more than 6 months.
Chasteberry (*Vitex agnus-castus*)	May counteract the effectiveness of birth control pills.
Ginkgo biloba (*Ginkgo biloba*)	Do not use with antidepressant MAO inhibitor drugs, such as phenelzine sulfate (Nardil) or tranylcypromine (Parnate); aspirin or other nonsteroidal anti-inflammatory medications; or blood-thinning medications such as warfarin (Coumadin). Can cause dermatitis, diarrhea, and vomiting in doses higher than 240 milligrams of concentrated extract.
Gymnema sylvestre (*Gymnema sylvestre*)	May influence blood sugar levels. Do not use without medical supervision if you have diabetes.
Kava kava (*Piper methysticum*)	Do not take with alcohol or barbiturates. Do not take more than the recommended dose on package. Use caution when driving or operating equipment because this herb is a muscle relaxant.
Lobelia (*Lobelia inflata*)	Can cause nausea and vomiting in large doses.
Periwinkle (*Vinca minor*)	Do not use if you have low blood pressure or constipation.
St. John's wort (*Hypericum perforatum*)	Do not use with antidepressants or other prescription medicine without medical approval. May cause photosensitivity; avoid overexposure to direct sunlight.
Stinging nettle (*Urtica dioica*)	If you have allergies, your symptoms may worsen, so take only one dose a day for the first few days.

Safe Use of Vitamins, Minerals, and Other Supplements

Although reports of toxicity from vitamins, minerals, and other supplements are rare, adverse reactions do happen. This guide is designed to alert you to some known reactions associated with some of the supplements described in this book. (The list covers only those supplements and is not comprehensive.)

For best absorption and minimal stomach irritation, take supplements with a meal unless otherwise directed. If you have a serious chronic illness that requires continual medical supervision, always discuss supplementation with your doctor. Similarly, if you are pregnant, nursing, or attempting to conceive, do not supplement without the supervision of your doctor.

Supplement	Safety Guidelines and Possible Side Effects
Acetyl-L-carnitine	Doses above 2,000 milligrams may cause mild diarrhea.
DHEA	Take only under the supervision of a knowledgeable naturopathic or medical professional. May cause liver damage, acne, irritability, irregular heart rhythms, accelerated growth of existing tumors, altered hormone profiles, increased cancer risk (prostate in men and breast in women), hair loss in men and women, and growth of facial hair and deepening of the voice in women. Men and women under 35 should avoid because it suppresses the body's natural production of DHEA.
Fish oil	Do not take if any of the following apply: bleeding disorder, uncontrolled high blood pressure, use of anticoagulants (blood thinners) or regular aspirin, allergy to any kind of fish. People with diabetes should not take fish oil because of its high fat content. Increases bleeding time, possibly resulting in nosebleeds and easy bruising. May cause stomach upset.
Folic acid	Excess folic acid from supplements can cause progressive nerve damage in individuals—usually older people—with vitamin B_{12} deficiency.
Glutamine	If you have problems with your kidneys or liver, check with your physician before supplementing.
L-lysine	Experimental. Long-term effects unknown. Don't take without a doctor's guidance. Don't take arginine and lysine at the same time because they compete for absorption in the body.
L-proline	Do not use without the guidance of a physician. Do not exceed dosages of 3,000 to 4,000 milligrams.
L-tyrosine	Do not take if you are on MAO inhibitor drugs because it can cause sweating and elevated blood pressure.
Melatonin	Causes drowsiness; take only at bedtime and never before driving. May cause headaches, nausea, morning dizziness, daytime sleepiness, depression, giddiness, difficulty concentrating, and upset stomach. May cause interactions with pre-

Supplement	Safety Guidelines and Possible Side Effects
	scription medications. Has adverse effects on people with any of the following: cardiovascular condition, high blood pressure, any autoimmune disease (such as rheumatoid arthritis or lupus), diabetes, epilepsy, migraine, or a personal or family history of a hormone-dependent cancer (such as breast, testicular, prostate, or endometrial). May cause infertility, reduced sex drive in males, hypothermia, retinal damage, and interference with hormone replacement therapy. Long-term effects of melatonin supplements are unknown.
SAM-e	May increase blood levels of homocysteine, a significant risk factor for cardiovascular disease.
Vitamin B$_6$	Taking more than 100 milligrams a day can cause reversible nerve damage. When selecting a B-complex supplement, check the label for the amount of each ingredient to help you determine its safe use.
Vitamin C	Taking more than 2,000 milligrams a day can cause diarrhea in some people. To help maintain levels of vitamin C throughout the day, take half of the recommended dose in the morning and half at night.
Vitamin D	Taking more than 2,000 international units (50 micrograms) a day can cause headache, fatigue, nausea, diarrhea, or loss of appetite.
Vitamin E	The safe upper limit from supplements only is 1,500 IU (natural form, d-alpha-tocopherol) or 1,100 IU (synthetic form, dl-alpha-tocopherol) a day. Because it acts as a blood thinner, consult your doctor before taking vitamin E if you are already taking aspirin or a blood-thinning medication, such as warfarin (Coumadin).

Index

Boldface page references indicate illustrations. Underscored references indicate boxed text.